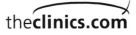

NURSING CLINICS

OF NORTH AMERICA

Biology, Psychology, and Behavior in Cardiovascular and Pulmonary Disease

GUEST EDITORS
Susan K. Frazier, PhD, RN
Terry A. Lennie, PhD, RN
Debra K. Moser, DNSc, RN, FAAN

CONSULTING EDITOR
Suzanne S. Prevost, PhD, RN

March 2008 • Volume 43 • Number 1

SAUNDERS

An Imprint of Elsevier, Inc.
PHILADELPHIA   LONDON   TORONTO   MONTREAL   SYDNEY   TOKYO

W.B. SAUNDERS COMPANY
A Division of Elsevier Inc.

1600 John F. Kennedy Blvd., Suite 1800, Philadelphia, PA 19103-2899

http://www.theclinics.com

NURSING CLINICS OF NORTH AMERICA Volume 43, Number 1
March 2008 ISSN 0029-6465
Editor: Ali Gavenda ISBN-13: 978-1-4160-5776-5
ISBN-10: 1-4160-5776-5

The ideas and opinions expressed in *Nursing Clinics of North America* do not necessarily reflect those of the Publisher. The Publisher does not assume any responsibility for any injury and/or damage to persons or property arising out of or related to any use of the material contained in this periodical. The reader is advised to check the appropriate medical literature and the product information currently provided by the manufacturer of each drug to be administered to verify the dosage, the method and duration of administration, or contraindications. It is the responsibility of the treating physician or other health care professional, relying on independent experience and knowledge of the patient, to determine drug dosages and the best treatment for the patient. Mention of any product in this issue should not be construed as endorsement by the contributors, editors, or the Publisher of the product or manufacturers' claims.

Nursing Clinics of North America (ISSN 0029-6465) is published quarterly by Elsevier Inc., 360 Park Avenue South, New York, NY 10010-1710. Months of issue are March, June, September, and December. Business and Editorial Offices: 1600 John F. Kennedy Blvd., Suite 1800, Philadelphia, PA 19103-2899. Customer Service Office: 6277 Sea Harbor Drive, Orlando, FL 32887-4800. Periodicals postage paid at New York, NY and additional mailing offices. Subscription price per year is, $123.00 (US individuals), $242.00 (US institutions), $198.00 (international individuals), $290.00 (international institutions), $170.00 (Canadian individuals), $290.00 (Canadian institutions), $65.00 (US students), and $100.00 (international students). To receive student/resident rate, orders must be accompanied by name of affiliated institution, date of term, and the signature of program/residency coordinator on institution letterhead. Orders will be billed at individual rate until proof of status is received. Foreign air speed delivery is included in all *Clinics* subscription prices. All prices are subject to change without notice. **POSTMASTER:** Send address changes to *Nursing Clinics*, Elsevier Periodicals Customer Service, 6277 Sea Harbor Drive, Orlando, FL 32887-4800. **Customer Service: 1-800-654-2452 (US). From outside the United States, call 1-407-563-6020. Fax: 1-407-363-9661. E-mail: JournalsCustomerService-usa@elsevier.com.**

Nursing Clinics of North America is covered in *EMBASE/Excerpta Medica, Index Medicus, Social Sciences Citation Index, Current Contents, ASCA, Cumulative Index to Nursing, RNdex Top 100,* and *Allied Health Literature and International Nursing Index (INI).*

Printed in the United States of America.

11/26/08

CONSULTING EDITOR

SUZANNE S. PREVOST, PhD, RN, Nursing Professor and National HealthCare Chair of Excellence, School of Nursing, Middle Tennessee State University, Murfreesboro, Tennessee

GUEST EDITORS

SUSAN K. FRAZIER, PhD, RN, Associate Professor, College of Nursing, University of Kentucky, Lexington, Kentucky

TERRY A. LENNIE, PhD, RN, Associate Professor, College of Nursing and Graduate Center for Nutritional Sciences, University of Kentucky, Lexington, Kentucky

DEBRA K. MOSER, DNSc, RN, FAAN, Professor and Gill Endowed Chair; Editor, Director, RICH Heart Program, The Journal of Cardiovascular Nursing, College of Nursing, University of Kentucky, Lexington, Kentucky

CONTRIBUTORS

GERENE S. BAULDOFF, PhD, RN, FCCP, Associate Professor of Clinical Nursing, College of Nursing, The Ohio State University, Columbus, Ohio

PATRICIA V. BURKHART, PhD, RN, Associate Professor, College of Nursing, University of Kentucky, Lexington, Kentucky

REBECCA L. DEKKER, MSN, RN, PhD student, College of Nursing, University of Kentucky, Lexington, Kentucky

SUSAN K. FRAZIER, PhD, RN, Associate Professor, College of Nursing, University of Kentucky, Lexington, Kentucky

FRANCES HARDIN-FANNING, RN, MSN, Lecturer, College of Nursing, University of Kentucky, Lexington, Kentucky

TRACI HOUSTEN-HARRIS, MS, RN, Pulmonary Hypertension Program, Johns Hopkins University, Baltimore, Maryland

LYNNE A. JENSEN, PhD, ARNP, BC, Assistant Clinical Professor, Director for Clinical Care, Center for the Advancement for Women's Health, College of Nursing, University of Kentucky, Lexington, Kentucky

DOROTHY S. LEE, MSN, APRN BC, PhD Candidate, College of Nursing, Wayne State University; and Research Nurse Practitioner, Respiratory Physiology Laboratory, John D. Dingell Veterans Affairs Medical Center, Detroit, Michigan

TERRY A. LENNIE, PhD, RN, Associate Professor, College of Nursing and Graduate Center for Nutritional Sciences, University of Kentucky, Lexington, Kentucky

DEBRA K. MOSER, DNSc, RN, FAAN, Professor and Gill Endowed Chair; Editor, Director, RICH Heart Program, The Journal of Cardiovascular Nursing, College of Nursing, University of Kentucky, Lexington, Kentucky

DAVID R. NUNLEY, MD, FCCP, Associate Professor of Clinical Medicine, Division of Pulmonary, Critical Care, and Sleep Medicine, The Ohio State University, Columbus, Ohio

HEATHER PAYNE-EMERSON, BS, RD, Doctoral Student, Graduate Center for Nutritional Sciences, University of Kentucky, Lexington, Kentucky

MI-KYUNG SONG, RN, PhD, Assistant Professor, Adult/Geriatric Health Division, School of Nursing, University of North Carolina, Chapel Hill, North Carolina

ANNETTE DE VITO DABBS, RN, PhD, Assistant Professor, Department of Acute & Tertiary Care, School of Nursing, University of Pittsburgh, Pittsburgh, Pennsylvania

JIA-RONG WU, PhD, RN, Post-doctoral Fellow, College of Nursing, University of Kentucky, Lexington, Kentucky; Lecturer, Department of Nursing, Chung Jung Christian University, Tainan, Taiwan

CONTENTS

Because of their anatomic position in the closed thoracic cavity, the heart and lungs interact during each ventilation cycle. The application of mechanical ventilation and subsequent removal changes normal ventilatory mechanics and produces alterations in cardiac preload and afterload that influence global hemodynamic state and delivery of oxygen and nutrients. Adverse cardiovascular responses to mechanical ventilation and weaning from ventilation include hemodynamic alterations and instability, myocardial ischemia, autonomic dysfunction, and cardiac dysrhythmias. Clinicians must have a clear understanding of the cardiovascular effects of mechanical ventilation and weaning so they may anticipate, recognize, and effectively manage negative effects and improve patient outcomes.

Pulmonary hypertension occurs when pulmonary vascular pressures are elevated. Pulmonary arterial hypertension is associated with occlusion of the pulmonary arterial tree, while pulmonary venous hypertension is seen when pulmonary vein outflow is impeded. Cardiovascular consequences are common with pulmonary hypertension, regardless of the underlying pathogenesis and whether management is complex. However, there are a number of interventions that may improve quality of life and survival of pulmonary hypertension. This article discusses current recommendations for diagnosis and management.

knowledgeable than men in the identification of risk factors and less common symptoms of AMI.

The Effects of a Mediterranean-Style Dietary Pattern on Cardiovascular Disease Risk

Frances Hardin-Fanning

Dietary patterns influence cardiovascular disease by inhibiting or promoting atherogenesis. Certain nutrients play key roles at different stages of this process, and the combined nutrients of a Mediterranean-style diet offer a significant source of primary and secondary disease prevention. Although current evidence does not support recommendations for or against single-nutrient supplementation, a Mediterranean-style diet should be recommended to reduce the risk of cardiovascular disease. Current nutrition recommendations and mechanisms by which a Mediterranean-style diet impacts cardiovascular risk are described in this article.

Nutritional Considerations in Heart Failure

Heather Payne-Emerson and Terry A. Lennie

There are a number of factors related to heart failure pathophysiology and treatment that influence nutrient requirements for patients. These include catabolism, inflammation, oxidative stress, diuretic use, and presence of comorbidities. On the other hand, there is evidence that specific nutrients can alter heart failure pathophysiology. This article reviews the current evidence for nutritional recommendations regarding sodium and fluid restriction, macro- and micronutrient intake, and dietary changes required by the presence of common comorbidities.

Medication Adherence in Patients Who Have Heart Failure: a Review of the Literature

Jia-Rong Wu, Debra K. Moser, Terry A. Lennie, and Patricia V. Burkhart

Data indicate that nonadherence plays a major role in preventable rehospitalizations. The first step to improving adherence is determining the affecting factor. This article critically reviews the literature on factors affecting medication adherence in heart failure patients. Findings about effects of age, gender, race, and living status on adherence are quite inconsistent. Patients who believe taking medications is beneficial or who have no side effects are more adherent, as are those highly motivated to improve their well-being. Forgetfulness, social support, and patient-provider relationship are related to adherence. Providers seeking to increase adherence must consider patients' expectations for their health, their environment, their barriers to following prescribed regimen, and their understanding of their condition and how it relates to medication taking.

Cognitive Behavioral Therapy for Depression in Patients with Heart Failure: A Critical Review
Rebecca L. Dekker

Depression is a significant problem in patients with heart failure. Cognitive behavioral therapy (CBT) has been proposed as a potential non-pharmacological treatment for depression in patients with heart failure. The purpose of this review is to examine the evidence for the use of CBT in treating depression and depressive symptoms in patients with cardiovascular illness. In six of the ten studied reviewed, researchers found that CBT reduced depressive symptoms; however, the limitations of the studies prevent wide generalization of the results. There is insufficient evidence to support the use of CBT for the treatment of depressive symptoms in patients with cardiovascular illness at this time. Large randomized, controlled trials that demonstrate the efficacy of CBT are needed before nurses routinely refer patients with heart failure to CBT for the purpose of improving depression or depressive symptoms.

FORTHCOMING ISSUES

RECENT ISSUES

NURSING
CLINICS
OF NORTH AMERICA

Nurs Clin N Am 43 (2008) xi–xii

ELSEVIER
SAUNDERS

Preface

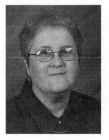
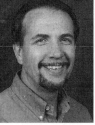
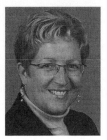

Susan K. Frazier,
PhD, RN

Terry A. Lennie,
PhD, RN
Guest Editors

Debra K. Moser,
DNSc, RN, FAAN

Virtually all cardiovascular and most pulmonary diseases are chronic in nature. Chronic cardiac or pulmonary diseases comprise three of the top four causes of death (ie, heart disease, cancers, stroke, and chronic lower respiratory diseases). Worldwide, cardiovascular disease (CVD) is the most common cause of death and morbidity, and in most developed countries is the single largest health care expenditure [1,2]. At least one in three Americans lives with chronic CVD; this percentage increases with age, and, ultimately, one in two dies of CVD, usually after living for years with the challenge of engaging in self-management of the chronic condition [1,2]. The World Health Organization estimates that chronic lower respiratory diseases share fourth and fifth places with HIV/AIDS as causes of death worldwide. In 2005, there were more than 3 million deaths worldwide from chronic obstructive pulmonary disease, which corresponds to 5% of all deaths globally [3].

The appropriate and effective management of cardiovascular and pulmonary diseases requires that nurses understand the complex interactions among the underlying pathophysiology, psychologic responses to the disease processes, and the behaviors that can improve or worsen illness trajectory. Current statistics elaborating the impact of chronic cardiovascular and pulmonary conditions [1,4] illustrate the importance of understanding these interactions. This issue of *Nursing Clinics of North America* provides an in-depth discussion of the physiologic cardiac and lung interactions in both cardiovascular and pulmonary diseases, the impact of psychologic and

doi:10.1016/j.cnur.2007.11.004   *nursing.theclinics.com* behavioral factors on cardiovascular disease, and the interplay among these factors. The specific topics covered in this issue have relevance across most chronic cardiovascular and pulmonary diseases. Collectively the articles provide a comprehensive understanding of the biologic, psychologic, and behavioral components that will be useful in the management of a variety of complex patient populations.

Susan K. Frazier, PhD, RN
College of Nursing
University of Kentucky
523 CON Building, 760 Rose Street
Lexington, KY 40536, USA

E-mail address: skfraz2@email.uky.edu

Terry A. Lennie, PhD, RN
College of Nursing
University of Kentucky
529 CON Building, 760 Rose Street
Lexington, KY 40536, USA

E-mail address: tlennie@uky.edu

Debra K. Moser, DNSc, RN, FAAN
College of Nursing
University of Kentucky
527 CON Building, 760 Rose Street
Lexington, KY 40536, USA

E-mail address: dmoser@uky.edu

References

[1] Rosamond W, Flegal K, Friday G, et al. Heart disease and stroke statistics—2007 update: a report from the American Heart Association Statistics Committee and Stroke Statistics Subcommittee. Circulation 2007;115(5):e69–171.
[2] Mensah GA, Brown DW. An overview of cardiovascular disease burden in the United States. Health Aff (Millwood) 2007;26(1):38–48.
[3] Lopez AD, Mathers CD, Ezzati M, et al. Global burden of disease and risk factors. Washington (DC): The World Bank; 2006.
[4] Prevalence of heart disease—United States, 2005. MMRW Morb Mortal Wkly Rep 2007; 56(6):113–8.

ELSEVIER
SAUNDERS

NURSING
CLINICS
OF NORTH AMERICA

Nurs Clin N Am 43 (2008) 1–15

Cardiovascular Effects of Mechanical Ventilation and Weaning

Susan K. Frazier, PhD, RN

College of Nursing, University of Kentucky, 523 CON Building, 760 Rose Street, Lexington, KY 40536-0232, USA

Mechanical ventilation is the most common support intervention used in critical care units and its use has increased an estimated 11% in recent years [1]. Thus, it is vital that clinicians have a clear understanding of the global effects of this intervention in order to provide safe and effective care to this escalating population. Mechanical ventilation supports acid base homeostasis, carbon dioxide removal, and adequate oxygenation in critically ill patients. Although mechanical ventilation is life supporting, there are a number of negative consequences associated with its use. These include the development of ventilator-associated pneumonia [2], pulmonary barotraumas [3], and malnutrition [4]. In addition, alterations in intrathoracic pressure and alveolar gas volume produced by mechanical ventilation may create profound cardiovascular effects because of the location of both heart and lungs in the closed thoracic cavity [5]. Cardiovascular alterations with mechanical ventilation may be detrimental or beneficial; global consequences depend on fundamental cardiac function and the adequacy of cardiovascular compensation [5–7].

Because of their anatomic position in the closed thoracic cavity, the heart and lungs interact during each ventilation cycle. During spontaneous ventilation, the results of this interaction are usually subtle; however, the institution of positive-pressure mechanical ventilation significantly alters ventilatory mechanics and may induce serious cardiovascular alterations. Positive-pressure ventilation generates positive intrathoracic pressure on inspiration (Fig. 1). This is in contrast to spontaneous inspiration, whereby a less than atmospheric intrathoracic pressure is produced by diaphragm contraction, a pressure gradient is formed between the atmosphere and the alveoli, and gas flows into the alveoli along the gradient. Gas flow continues until the pressure difference reaches zero (end-inspiration).

E-mail address: skfraz2@email.uky.edu

0029-6465/08/$ - see front matter © 2008 Elsevier Inc. All rights reserved.
doi:10.1016/j.cnur.2007.10.001

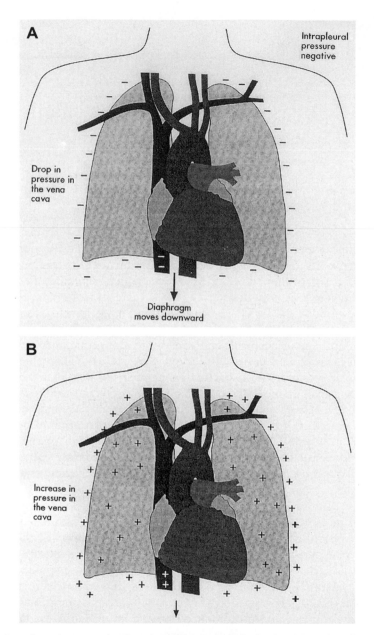

Fig. 1. Intrathoracic pressure is reflected upon the structures in the closed thoracic cavity and may influence venous return because of a number of mechanisms. (*A*) Intrathoracic pressure during spontaneous ventilation is less than atmospheric (−). Venous return is increased with inspiration because of augmentation in the venous return pressure gradient. (*B*) Intrathoracic pressure during mechanical ventilation is positive (+). Venous return is reduced due to compression of the pliable vena cava and increase in right ventricular afterload. (*From* Pilbeam SP. Mechanical ventilation. Physiological and clinical application. 3rd ed. St. Louis (MO): Mosby; 1998; with permission.)

Diaphragm relaxation then reduces the size of the thoracic cavity, increases intrathoracic pressure, and generates a pressure gradient for gas flow out of the alveoli. Gas flow continues outward until the pressure difference reaches zero (end-expiration) and the cycle begins again. During mechanical ventilation, gas is delivered during inspiration using some degree of pressure as the driving force.

Common modes of mechanical ventilation are volume and/or pressure-controlled and typically produce varying degrees of positive intrathoracic pressure during inspiration. Less commonly used modes of ventilation, such as inverse ratio ventilation, produce prolonged positive intrathoracic pressure during a prolonged inspiratory period. Administration of positive end-expiratory pressure (PEEP) or the use of continuous positive airway pressure (CPAP) intend to increase functional residual capacity and improve oxygenation. However, intrathoracic pressure remains positive throughout the entire ventilatory cycle when these are used. The alterations in ventilatory mechanics inherent to the use of mechanical ventilation generate changes in cardiac preload and afterload that influence global hemodynamic state and delivery of oxygen and nutrients.

Right heart effects of positive-pressure ventilation

During inspiration, the positive intrathoracic pressure produced by a mechanical breath decreases venous return. An increase in intrathoracic pressure as small as 4 mm Hg is associated with a reduction in venous return by 50% for a transient period of time [8]. In individuals with normal cardiac function, venous return and subsequent cardiac output may be dramatically reduced with the institution of mechanical ventilation, particularly in individuals with coexisting hypovolemia or states that produce systemic vasodilation or relative hypovolemia, like septic shock [9]. Cardiac output and mean arterial pressure may precipitously decrease following initiation of mechanical ventilation; this reduction may be dramatic and require emergent attention. In most instances, the consequences of reduced venous return are alleviated by intravenous fluid administration and adequate augmentation of blood volume [9]. Inherent compensation for this hemodynamic response is produced by a complex neurohormonal response that includes catecholamine release and secretion of arginine vasopressin and renin with subsequent increases in angiotensin II and aldosterone [10]. Natriuretic peptide hormone secretion is reduced with less cardiac chamber volume to stimulate hormone release. The net effect of these responses is sodium and water retention to support adequate preload and vasoconstriction to increase blood pressure.

Patients with heart failure may actually improve cardiac function with the application of mechanical ventilation, in part because of this reduction in venous return [11,12]. Unless optimally managed, patients with heart failure have a chronic increase in preload because of persistent stimulation of the renin angiotensin aldosterone system, reduction in natriuretic peptide release, and secretion of arginine vasopressin. Patients with heart failure also exhibit a perpetually elevated systemic vascular resistance partly because of chronic sympathetic nervous system activation. Application of mechanical ventilation reduces venous return and moderates the ventricular volume load. This reduced volume load will decrease ventricular wall tension and support the mechanical efficiency of the heart. Thus, in patients with heart failure, cardiac function may dramatically improve with the application of mechanical ventilation.

The mechanisms that produce this response are complex and not completely understood. The pressure gradient for venous return develops between right atrial pressure and mean systemic pressure. Flow to the right atrium will cease when these pressures are equal [13]. However, intrathoracic pressure changes associated with mechanical ventilation have been found to increase right atrial pressure and systemic mean pressure equally. Thus, the reductions in venous return are primarily independent of changes in this pressure gradient [14]. Positive intrathoracic pressure compresses the compliant vena cava and increases resistance to venous flow. The vena cava may collapse intermittently and obliterate flow with sufficiently increased intrathoracic pressure.

Pulmonary vascular resistance and right ventricular output impedance, indicators of right ventricular afterload, are augmented during the mechanical ventilation inspiratory cycle. With the addition of PEEP or CPAP, afterload may be increased throughout the ventilatory cycle [15–17]. The vascular resistance of alveolar vessels increases as alveoli expand with gas, and vessel compression occurs as alveoli inflate; thus, tidal volume is the primary determinant of right ventricular afterload [15–17]. Augmentation in right ventricular afterload necessitates the right ventricle generate greater pressure to eject blood into the pulmonary artery. Accordingly, right ventricular work and myocardial oxygen demands are increased.

Nutritive blood flow to the right ventricle is approximately equal during systole and diastole in normal coronary arteries [8,18]. The pressure gradient that produces coronary blood flow is developed between the root of the aorta at the coronary ostia and the arterioles located within the right ventricular myocardium. An increase in right ventricular intrachamber pressure or end-diastolic volume may reduce this pressure gradient for coronary blood flow and potentially decrease flow and myocardial oxygen delivery at a time when oxygen demand is increased. This is more likely to occur in individuals who require mechanical ventilation and have concomitant coronary artery disease. Significant reductions in coronary artery flow in these individuals produce myocardial ischemia and subsequent abnormalities in wall motion like hypokinesis and dyskinesis. These influence cardiac pumping ability, which in turn will further reduce ejection fraction, increase end-diastolic volume, and worsen coronary flow. Myocardial infarction may be the ultimate consequence.

Individuals who are unable to sufficiently increase contractile force in response to increased right ventricular afterload have a subsequent reduction in right ventricular stroke volume and ejection fraction. The resultant increase in end-diastolic volume dilates the right ventricle. Ventricular dilation will alter the pressure gradient for coronary artery blood flow, increase ventricular wall tension, and shift the interventricular septum toward the left ventricle [19]. Subsequently, left ventricular chamber size and compliance will be reduced and left ventricular filling impeded (Fig. 2). Thus, left ventricular function may be significantly altered by right ventricular effects of mechanical ventilation.

Left heart effects of positive-pressure ventilation

Several of the left ventricular effects of mechanical ventilation are directly attributed to alterations in right ventricular function, particularly the effects on left ventricular preload or end-diastolic volume [5]. Reduced venous return subsequently decreases the volume of blood the left ventricle receives. Thus, left ventricular preload is decreased and subsequent stroke volume and cardiac output are less. Increased right ventricular afterload and right ventricular dilation with shift of the interventricular septum reduces left ventricular chamber size, compliance, and filling, which also leads to reduced left ventricular preload [19]. Left ventricular preload may also be influenced by increased pericardial pressure [20]. Hyperinflated lungs directly compress the heart, reduce cardiac compliance, and lessen ventricular filling and end-diastolic volumes. These responses to mechanical ventilation all reduce left ventricular preload.

Positive pressure mechanical ventilation also reduces left ventricular afterload or transmural pressure on inspiration and throughout the ventilatory cycle with the application of PEEP or CPAP [5,6]. Transmural pressure is the pressure inside the ventricular chamber minus pressure outside the ventricle (intrathoracic pressure). Left ventricular transmural pressure is an indication of the pressure the ventricle must overcome to eject blood into the aorta. Positive intrathoracic pressure actually unloads the left ventricle by reducing transmural pressure. Consequently, the left ventricle is able to eject a greater stroke volume of blood with less pressure generation. Thus, myocardial oxygen demand is reduced and cardiac output improves. Patients with heart failure particularly benefit from mechanical ventilation by significantly increasing cardiac output with less myocardial oxygen consumption because of the combination of a reduction in ventricular volumes and a decrease in left ventricular afterload [13,14].

Cardiovascular effects of ventilator weaning

There have been a number of reports of the cardiovascular effects of the return to spontaneous ventilation after a period of mechanical ventilation

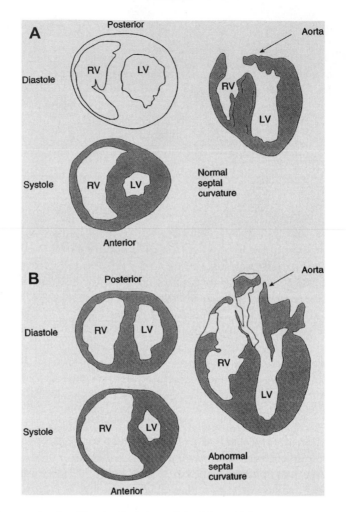

Fig. 2. Cross-sectional and longitudinal views of the right and left ventricle and interventricular septum during systole and diastole. (*A*) Normal relationship between ventricles. (*B*) Dilation of the right ventricle with shift of the interventricular septum toward the left ventricle. (*From* Darovic GO. Hemodynamic monitoring. Invasive and noninvasive clinical application. 3rd ed. Philadelphia (PA): Saunders; 2002; with permission.)

[7,21–25]. This action is referred to as "ventilator weaning" even though a majority of patients do not require the gradual reduction in support implied [26]. A variety of weaning modes have been developed that provide varying levels of mechanical support to ease this transition and improve the likelihood of success. Their effect on cardiovascular function is dependent upon the changes generated in intrathoracic pressure and lung volume and on fundamental cardiac function [5–7].

A number of studies have evaluated mechanisms that produced weaning failure in a variety of intensive care populations. In an early study, Demling and colleagues [27] found that approximately one third of a group of surgical and burn patients failed to successfully institute independent ventilation when they developed acute heart failure; another group of investigators [28] found that about 25% of their medical intensive care unit patients who failed to wean from ventilation also developed acute heart failure. Later investigations found that patients with left ventricular dysfunction required significantly more ventilator days in comparison with patients who had normal cardiac function [29,30]. Other investigators [31] found that the presence of severe left ventricular dysfunction predicted extubation failure in cardiac surgery patients. The need for intropic support, the use of an intra-aortic balloon pump, and the presence of atrial arrhythmias were found to be significant risk factors for delayed extubation in patients ventilated after coronary artery bypass surgery [32]. More recently, patients who required long-term mechanical ventilation following cardiac surgery were nearly 11 times more likely to fail ventilator weaning when their left ventricular ejection fraction was less than 40% (odds ratio [OR] 10.56, $P < .001$) [33]. Identified adverse cardiovascular responses to ventilator weaning include hemodynamic alterations and instability, myocardial ischemia, autonomic dysfunction, and cardiac dysrhythmias (Fig. 3).

Hemodynamic alterations

The return to spontaneous ventilation and normal mechanics of ventilation produces significant hemodynamic alterations that generate an abrupt increase in venous return and left ventricular afterload. Should hypoventilation and alveolar hypoxia occur, hypoxic pulmonary vasoconstriction ensues and contributes to increases in pulmonary vascular resistance and right ventricular afterload [17,34]. Hypoxic pulmonary vasoconstriction, a compensatory response that intends to better match ventilation and perfusion, may significantly impede right ventricular ejection and produce right ventricular dilation, reduced coronary blood flow, and shift of the interventricular septum into the left ventricle [5,6]. In addition, the immediate increase in left ventricular transmural pressure and afterload may hinder left ventricular ejection and result in an increase in left ventricular end-diastolic volume and pressure. Left ventricular dilation, increased wall stress, and acute heart failure and pulmonary edema may follow. Reductions in coronary blood flow may also occur.

Beach and colleagues [21] published one of the first reports of hemodynamic alterations during ventilator weaning and identified differential cardiovascular responses to ventilator weaning in a group of postoperative cardiac surgical patients (n = 37). Slightly more than half the patients increased cardiac output by an average of 19% in response to spontaneous ventilation; the remaining patients reduced cardiac output by an average of 17% with spontaneous ventilation. Patients who reduced cardiac output also demonstrated an increase in pulmonary and systemic vascular resistance

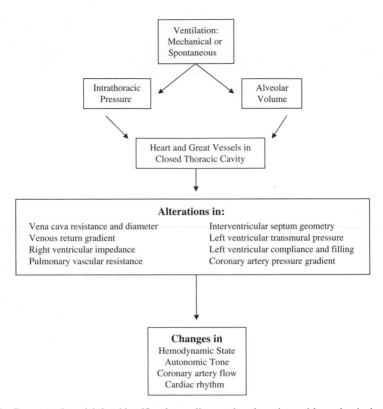

Fig. 3. Conceptual model that identifies the cardiovascular alterations with mechanical ventilation and ventilator weaning. Ventilation, either mechanical or spontaneous, produces alterations in intrathoracic pressure and alveolar volume, which are reflected on the heart and great vessels. A number of cardiovascular changes result that may produce hemodynamic instability, autonomic dysfunction, myocardial ischemia, and cardiac rhythm disturbances.

and central venous pressure. Since that seminal publication, other investigators have identified increased right ventricular end-diastolic volume [30], reduced cardiac output [23,25], elevated pulmonary artery pressures and pulmonary vascular resistance [22,23], greater left ventricular filling pressures [24], and an increased prevalence of left ventricular dilation in response to ventilator weaning in patients who failed to sustain independent spontaneous ventilation after a period of mechanical ventilation [24].

Weaning modes that provide some level of mechanical support during the process may reduce hemodynamic alterations. Richard and colleagues [24] found that left ventricular ejection fraction significantly decreased during spontaneous ventilation, but there was no significant change seen during pressure support weaning in a group of chronic obstructive pulmonary disease patients without coronary artery disease. Raper and Sibbald [35] found that incremental CPAP significantly and progressively increased pulmonary vascular resistance and reduced right ventricular ejection fraction as CPAP level increased. Frazier and colleagues [7] found that spontaneous ventilation with CPAP and T-piece weaning significantly increased right ventricular stroke work and oxygen demand, while pressure support did not alter the required work. Most of these investigators concluded that different weaning modes alter cardiovascular performance, but global consequences depend on the efficacy of cardiovascular compensatory mechanisms.

Several recent studies have evaluated plasma B-type natriuretic peptide (BNP) concentration as a biomarker of left ventricular dysfunction in ventilated patients. BNP, a hormone released by cardiac myocytes in response to myocardial wall stretch, produces natriuretic and diuretic effects. In a recent study [36], elevated BNP concentration nearly doubled the likelihood of weaning failure (OR 1.9, $P < .001$). In this investigation of medical intensive care patients (n = 112), slightly more than 40% failed to successfully wean from ventilation. Patients with a BNP concentration of 275 pg/mL or more required significantly longer duration of ventilation and longer weaning duration, and exhibited a significantly higher mortality rate ($P < .01$). BNP concentration of 275 pg/mL or more had a diagnostic accuracy of 86% for weaning failure in these patients. Another group of investigators [37] identified increased BNP concentrations during mechanical ventilation in medical intensive care patients who subsequently failed weaning. Both right and left ventricular dysfunction were identified in these patients using echocardiography. BNP concentration further increased in response to weaning; increases were greater in patients who exhibited left ventricular dysfunction compared with those who had right ventricular dysfunction. Preliminary studies suggest that BNP may be a useful biomarker in patients receiving mechanical ventilation.

Myocardial ischemia

Myocardial ischemia during ventilation and weaning may be the consequence of inadequate coronary blood flow produced by ventricular dilation, increased wall stress, and alterations in the pressure gradient for coronary blood flow. In the first reported study of ischemia during ventilator weaning, Hurford and colleagues [38] identified reductions in myocardial perfusion and dilation of the left ventricle in nearly half of a group of patients during weaning. Subsequently, Hurford and Favorito [39] demonstrated ST segment changes indicative of ischemia in 35% of a group of medical and surgical patients during weaning. Later, Abalos and colleagues [40] found that approximately 20% of a group of non-cardiac surgical patients exhibited ST segment changes indicative of ischemia, primarily during ventilator weaning. Another group of investigators measured myocardial lactate production in coronary artery bypass graft patients during ventilator weaning [41]. Even though these patients had recently undergone successful coronary revascularization, nearly half experienced ischemia during weaning as demonstrated by lactate production.

Myocardial ischemia has been found to approximately double the likelihood of weaning failure. Chatila and colleagues [42] found that about 6% of their medical and cardiac intensive care patients exhibited ischemic changes during weaning, but those who did were nearly twice as likely to fail to wean (relative risk 1.8). In a follow-up study, Srivastava and colleagues [43] identified ischemia in 10% of ventilated patients who had known coronary artery disease; these patients were again twice as likely to fail to wean (relative risk 2.1). More recently, Frazier and colleagues [44] studied medical intensive care patients during a period of mechanical ventilation and found that 56% displayed ischemic ST segment changes during ventilation; 16% of these patients also exhibited ischemia during ventilator weaning. Those patients who demonstrated ischemia during mechanical ventilation were 60% more likely to fail to wean successfully (relative risk 1.6).

Autonomic dysfunction

Compensatory responses to the hemodynamic changes induced by mechanical ventilation and weaning are produced to some extent by the autonomic nervous system. Interaction between sympathetic and parasympathetic stimulation normally produces beat-by-beat alterations in heart rate with subsequent changes in heart rate, vascular resistance, ventricular filling time, and ventricular contractility. This balance may be evaluated by analyses of the R-R intervals on the electrocardiogram or measures of heart rate variability [45]. Increased heart rate variability indicates parasympathetic dominance of cardiac control and because of positive action potential effects, increased electrical stability. Reduced heart rate variability is found with sympathetic dominance and negative effects on the action potential result (decreased ventricular refractoriness, increased electrical excitability).

Reduced heart rate variability was associated with worse outcomes in several patient populations. Reduced heart rate variability and autonomic dysfunction have been demonstrated in patients after acute myocardial infarction [46], following severe traumatic brain injury [47], in postoperative aortic surgery patients [48], in those with multiple organ dysfunction syndrome [49], and in patients with coronary artery disease [50] and heart failure [51,52]. Greater morbidity and mortality were strongly associated with reductions in heart rate variability in these studies, and in many instances, reduced heart rate variability was an independent predictor of negative outcomes.

Inappropriate autonomic responses to ventilator weaning were first described by Frazier and colleagues [52] in a laboratory animal study comparing autonomic responses to spontaneous ventilation with pressure support, continuous positive airway pressure, and a combination of the two modes. The combination of modes produced a reduction in heart rate variability suggesting sympathetic dominance occurred in response to this weaning mode. There were simultaneous reductions in right ventricular end-diastolic volume and increased heart rate. This combination of weaning modes significantly altered intrathoracic pressure and reduced venous return. Sympathetic neural outflow increased in response to these hemodynamic alterations and heart rate increased to maintain adequate cardiac output.

In a later study, Shen and colleagues [53] reported that a small group of ventilated patients who failed weaning reduced heart rate variability in response to a spontaneous breathing trial. In a study of medical intensive care patients, Frazier and colleagues [54] recently demonstrated reduced heart rate variability in a group of ventilated patients with high severity of illness (mean APACHE II score 26 ± 9). Those patients who failed their initial spontaneous breathing trial further reduced heart rate variability in response to the trial. Plasma norepinephrine concentrations also significantly increased in this group of patients supporting the increase in sympathetic stimulation. All these patients demonstrated some degree of autonomic dysfunction, but those who failed their initial weaning trial had a greater degree of dysfunction before and with the return to spontaneous ventilation.

Cardiac dysrhythmias

Because alterations in the balance between sympathetic and parasympathetic control of heart rate significantly influence cardiac action potentials, cardiac rhythm disturbances may be produced in response to ventilator weaning. Sympathetic stimulation has positive chronotropic and inotropic effects, which enhance automaticity, reduce refractory periods, augment excitability, and increase the probability of dysrhythmias. In addition, acute and chronic cardiac mechanical changes that occur with increases in chamber volume have been determined to be arrhythmogenic [55,56]. This mechano-electrical interaction response is likely a result of mechanical conformational changes in mechano-sensitive, ion-selective channels located in cardiac myocytes. Alterations in cytosolic ion concentrations that occur in response to these mechanical changes may induce dysrhythmias when action potential changes occur.

Frazier and colleagues [25] recently reported different patterns of ectopy in patients who were unable to establish independent spontaneous ventilation. Although all patients exhibited ventricular and supraventricular ectopy, ventricular ectopic beats per hour were reduced with spontaneous ventilation in those patients who were successfully weaned, while those who continued to require mechanical ventilation demonstrated no change in ventricular ectopy. All patients increased supraventricular ectopic beats in response to spontaneous ventilation, most likely because of mechano-electrical interaction. To date, the effect of ectopy on weaning outcome has not been evaluated.

Nursing implications

The application of positive-pressure mechanical ventilation may provoke significant hemodynamic response in critically ill patients. This is particularly true in patients with hypovolemia and those with heart failure. Individuals with hypovolemia will have negative responses, while those with heart failure may significantly improve with the application of mechanical ventilation. Clinicians must understand and anticipate these responses so that effective management is quickly instituted when required. Once ventilation is established and the patient stabilized, cardiovascular status should be carefully evaluated with each change in ventilator setting, particularly changes in those parameters that alter alveolar volume and/or intrathoracic pressure like PEEP level.

In patients who decrease cardiac output in response to positive intrathoracic pressure, activation of compensatory mechanisms like the renin angiotensin aldosterone system should be assumed. Thus, fluid volume status must be carefully monitored and evaluated. Fluid volume overload may occur in patients receiving ventilation, but not be obvious until the patient attempts to breathe spontaneously. Sympathetic nervous system activation must also be assumed with a resultant increase in systemic vascular resistance to some degree. Other effects of adrenergic stimulation must also be monitored and evaluated. These include increases in heart rate and contractility with concomitant increased myocardial oxygen requirement. Thus, the likelihood for silent myocardial ischemia should be considered for all patients receiving mechanical ventilation.

The re-institution of spontaneous ventilation is a time of hemodynamic change, regardless of the weaning mode used. Clinicians must consider cardiovascular status when determining readiness to wean from ventilation. Currently, most weaning protocols state only that patients should be "hemodynamically stable" without clear description of what that entails. However, without adequate cardiac function, sufficient oxygen delivery will not occur and weaning failure will ensue. Careful attention to cardiovascular state must also accompany weaning trials, particularly in those patients with a positive fluid balance. The return to spontaneous ventilation in the presence of hypervolemia can produce acute heart failure within minutes. Morbid events like cardiac dysrhythmias, myocardial ischemia, and pulmonary edema increase the likelihood of mortality in this vulnerable population. Appropriate monitoring with vigilant attention to cardiovascular state, early recognition of cardiovascular issues, and appropriate and effective intervention are mandatory to improve patient outcomes.

Summary

The application of mechanical ventilation increases intrathoracic pressure and alveolar gas volume, which alters cardiovascular state because of changes in preload and afterload. The return to spontaneous ventilation after a period of mechanical ventilation also induces cardiovascular changes. The global response to these alterations depends on the adequacy of cardiovascular compensatory mechanisms. Clinicians must have a clear understanding of the cardiovascular effects of ventilation and weaning so they may recognize and effectively manage negative effects and improve patient outcomes.

References

[1] Carson SS, Cox CE, Holmes GM, et al. The changing epidemiology of mechanical ventilation: a population-based study. J Intensive Care Med 2006;21(3):173–82.

[2] Combes A, Luyt CE, Fagon JY, et al. Early predictors for infection recurrence and death in patients with ventilator-associated pneumonia. Crit Care Med 2007;35(1):146–54.

[3] Gajic O, Frutos-Vivar F, Esteban A, et al. Ventilator settings as a risk factor for acute respiratory distress syndrome in mechanically ventilated patients. Intensive Care Med 2005;31: 922–6.

[4] Huang YC, Yen CE, Cheng CH, et al. Nutritional status of mechanically ventilated critically ill patients: comparison of different types of nutritional support. Clin Nutr 2000;19(2):101–7.

[5] Pinsky MR. Cardiovascular issues in respiratory care. Chest 2005;128(5):592S–7S.

[6] Steingrub JS, Tidswell M, Higgins TL. Hemodynamic consequences of heart-lung interactions. J Intensive Care Med 2003;18(2):92–9.

[7] Frazier SK, Stone KS, Schertel ER, et al. A comparison of hemodynamic changes during the transition from mechanical ventilation to T-piece, PS and CPAP in canines. Biol Res Nurs 2000;1(4):253–64.

[8] Dries D, Mathru M. Right ventricle: the neglected neighbor of the left. Austin (TX): R.G. Landes; 1994.

[9] Ramamoorthy C, Rooney M, Dries D, et al. Aggressive hydration during continuous positive-pressure ventilation restores atrial transmural pressure, plasma atrial natriuretic peptide concentrations, and renal function. Crit Care Med 1992;20:1014–9.

[10] Frazier SK. Neurohormonal responses during positive pressure mechanical ventilation. Heart Lung 1999;28(3):149–65.

[11] Javaheri S. Effects of continuous positive airway pressure on sleep apnea and ventricular irritability in patients with heart failure. Circulation 2000;101:392–7.

[12] Bradley TD, Logan AG, Kimoff RJ, et al. Continuous positive airway pressure for central sleep apnea and heart failure. N Engl J Med 2005;353(19):2025–33.

[13] Murphy BA, Durbin CG. Using ventilator and cardiovascular graphics in the patient who is hemodynamically unstable. Respir Care 2005;50(2):262–74.

[14] Jellinek H, Krenn H, Oczenski W, et al. Influence of positive airway pressure on the pressure gradient for venous return in humans. J Appl Physiol 2000;88:926–32.

[15] Koganov Y, Weiss YG, Oppenheim A, et al. Positive end-expiratory pressure increases pulmonary venous vascular resistance in patients after coronary artery surgery. Crit Care Med 1997;25(5):767–72.

[16] Jardin F, Vieillard-Baron A. Right ventricular function and positive pressure ventilation in clinical practice: from hemodynamic subsets to respirator settings. Intensive Care Med 2003; 29:1426–34.

[17] Viellard-Barton A, Loubieres Y, Schmitt JM, et al. Cyclic changes in right ventricular output impedance during mechanical ventilation. J Appl Physiol 1999;87(5):1644–50.

[18] Schulman D, Biondi, Zohgbi S, et al. Coronary flow limits right ventricular performance during positive end-expiratory pressure. Am Rev Respir Dis 1990;141:1531–7.

[19] Mitchell JR, Whitelaw WA, Sas R, et al. RV filling modulates LV function by direct ventricular interaction during mechanical ventilation. Am J Physiol Heart Circ Physiol 2005;289: H549–57.

[20] Fessler H, Brower R, Wise R, et al. Positive pleural pressure decreases coronary perfusion. Am J Physiol 1990;258(3):H814–20.

[21] Beach T, Millen E, Grenvik A. Hemodynamic response to discontinuance of mechanical ventilation. Crit Care Med 1973;1:85–90.

[22] Teboul J, Abrouk F, Lemaire F. Right ventricular function in COPD patients during weaning from mechanical ventilation. Intensive Care Med 1988;14:483–5.

[23] Lemaire F, Teboul J, Cinotti L, et al. Acute left ventricular dysfunction during unsuccessful weaning from mechanical ventilation. Anesthesiology 1988;69:171–9.

[24] Richard C, Teboul J, Archambaud F, et al. Left ventricular function during weaning of patients with chronic obstructive pulmonary disease. Intensive Care Med 1994;20:181–6.

[25] Frazier SK, Stone KS, Moser DK, et al. Hemodynamic changes during ventilator discontinuation in MICU patients. Am J Crit Care 2006;15(6):580–94.

[26] MacIntyre NR. Evidence-based guidelines for weaning and discontinuing ventilatory support: a collective task force facilitated by the American College of Chest Physicians; the American Association for Respiratory Care; and the American College of Critical Care Medicine. Chest 2001;120:375–96.

[27] Demling R, Read T, Lind L, et al. Incidence and morbidity of extubation failure in surgical intensive care patients. Crit Care Med 1988;16:573–7.

[28] Cheng DC, Peniston C, Asokumar B, et al. Morbidity outcome in early versus conventional tracheal extubation after coronary artery bypass grafting: a prospective randomized controlled trial. J Thorac Cardiovasc Surg 1996;112(3):755–64.

[29] Clochesy J, Daly B, Montenegro H. Weaning chronically critically ill adults from mechanical ventilatory support: a descriptive study. Am J Crit Care 1995;4:93–9.

[30] Sereika S, Clochesy J. Left ventricular dysfunction and duration of mechanical ventilatory support in the chronically critically ill: a survival analysis. Heart Lung 1996;25:45–51.

[31] Rady MY, Ryan T. Perioperative predictors of extubation failure and the effect on clinical outcome after cardiac surgery. Crit Care Med 1999;27(2):340–7.

[32] Wong DT, Cheng DC, Justra R, et al. Risk factors of delayed extubation, prolonged length of stay in the intensive care unit, and mortality in patients undergoing coronary artery bypass graft with fast-track cardiac anesthesia: a new cardiac risk score. Anesthesiology 1999;91(4):936–44.

[33] Nozawa E, Azeka E, Ignez M, et al. Factors associated with failure of weaning from long-term mechanical ventilation after cardiac surgery. Int Heart J 2005;80(3):301–10.

[34] Tsai BM, Wang M, Turrentine MW, et al. Hypoxic pulmonary vasoconstriction in cardiothoracic surgery: basic mechanisms to potential therapies. Ann Thorac Surg 2004;78:360–8.

[35] Raper R, Sibbald W. Increased right ventricular compliance in response to continuous positive airway pressure. Am Rev Respir Dis 1992;145:771–5.

[36] Mekontso-Dessap A, de Prost N, Girou E, et al. B-type natriuretic peptide and weaning from mechanical ventilation. Intensive Care Med 2006;32:1529–36.

[37] Ait-Oufella H, Tharaux PL, Baudel JL, et al. Variation in natriuretic peptides and mitral flow indexes during successful ventilatory weaning: a preliminary study. Intensive Care Med 2007;33(7):1183–6.

[38] Hurford W, Lynch K, Strauss H, et al. Myocardial perfusion as assessed by Thallium-201 scintigraphy during the discontinuation of mechanical ventilation in ventilator-dependent patients. Anesthesiology 1991;74:1007–16.

[39] Hurford W, Favorito F. Association of myocardial ischemia with failure to wean from mechanical ventilation. Crit Care Med 1995;23:1475–80.

[40] Abalos A, Leibowitz A, Distefano D, et al. Myocardial ischemia during the weaning period. Am J Crit Care 1992;3:32–6.

[41] Elia S, Liu P, Hilgenberg A, et al. Coronary haemodynamics and myocardial metabolism during weaning from mechanical ventilation in cardiac surgical patients. Can J Anaesth 1991;38:564–71.

[42] Chatila W, Ani S, Guaglianone D, et al. Cardiac ischemia during weaning from mechanical ventilation. Chest 1996;109:1577–83.

[43] Srivastava S, Chatila W, Amoateng-Adjepong Y, et al. Myocardial ischemia and weaning failure in patients with coronary artery disease: an update. Crit Care Med 1999;27:2109–12.

[44] Frazier SK, Brom H, Widener J, et al. The prevalence of myocardial ischemia during mechanical ventilation and weaning and its effects on weaning success. Heart Lung 2006; 35(6):363–73.

[45] Task Force of the European Society of Cardiology and the North American Society of Pacing and Electrophysiology. Heart rate variability. Standards of measurement, physiological interpretation, and clinical use. Circulation 1996;93(5):1043–65.

[46] La Rovere MT, Bigger JT, Marcus FI, et al. Baroreflex sensitivity and heart-rate variability in prediction of total cardiac mortality after myocardial infarction. Lancet 1998;351:478–84.

[47] Winchell RJ, Hoyt DB. Analysis of heart-rate variability: a noninvasive predictor of death and poor outcome in patients with severe head injury. J Trauma 1997;43(6):1108–9.

[48] Stein PK, Schmieg RE, El-Fouly A, et al. Association between heart rate variability recorded on postoperative day 1 and length of stay in abdominal aortic surgery patients. Crit Care Med 2001;29(9):1738–43.

[49] Schmidt H, Muller-Werdan U, Hoffmann T, et al. Autonomic dysfunction predicts mortality in patients with multiple organ dysfunction syndrome of different age groups. Crit Care Med 2005;31:1994–2002.

[50] van Boven AJ, Crijns HJ, Haaksma J, et al. Depressed heart rate variability is associated with events in patients with stable coronary artery disease and preserved left ventricular function. Am Heart J 1998;135(4):571–6.

[51] Galinier M, Parthak A, Fourcade J, et al. Depressed low frequency power of heart rate variability as an independent predictor of sudden death in chronic heart failure. Eur Heart J 2000;21:475–82.

[52] Frazier SK, Moser DK, Stone KS. Heart rate variability and hemodynamic alterations in canines with normal cardiac function during exposure to PS, CPAP and combination PS/ CPAP. Biol Res Nurs 2001;2(3):167–74.

[53] Shen HN, Lin LY, Chen KY, et al. Changes of heart rate variability during ventilator weaning. Chest 2003;123(4):1222–8.

[54] Frazier SK, Moser DK, Schlanger R, et al. Autonomic tone in medical intensive care patients receiving mechanical ventilation and during a CPAP weaning trial. Biol Res Nurs, in press.

[55] Franz MR. Mechano-electrical feedback. Circ Res 2000;45:263–6.

[56] Furukawa T, Ono Y, Tsuchiya H, et al. Specific interaction of the potassium channel b-subunit ink with the sarcomeric protein T-cap suggests a T-tubule-myofibril linking system. J Mol Biol 2001;313:775–84.

NURSING
CLINICS
OF NORTH AMERICA

Nurs Clin N Am 43 (2008) 17–36

Cardiovascular Consequences of Pulmonary Hypertension

Gerene S. Bauldoff, PhD, RN, FCCP[a],*,
Traci Housten-Harris, MS, RN[b],
David R. Nunley, MD, FCCP[c]

[a]*College of Nursing, The Ohio State University, 1585 Neil Avenue,
Columbus, OH 43210, USA*
[b]*Pulmonary Hypertension Program, Johns Hopkins University,
1830 East Monument Street, 5th Floor, Baltimore, MD 21205, USA*
[c]*Division of Pulmonary, Critical Care and Sleep Medicine, The Ohio State University,
201 Davis Heart & Lung Research Institute, 473 West 12th Avenue,
Columbus, OH 43210, USA*

Pulmonary hypertension (PH) is exemplified by elevated pulmonary arterial pressure and can be either idiopathic or arise secondary to a myriad of causes. Normal pulmonary artery pressure is 15 mm Hg to 20 mm Hg systolic and 8 mm Hg to 15 mm Hg diastolic. According to the National Heart, Lung, and Blood Institute (NHLBI) of the National Institutes of Health, pulmonary arterial hypertension (PAH) is defined as a mean pulmonary artery pressure greater than 25 mm Hg, with a pulmonary capillary or left atrial pressure of less than 15 mm Hg [1]. Developed in 1998 and updated in 2003, the World Health Organization (WHO) established a classification system for pulmonary hypertension [2] that includes five categories (Box 1). Use of the classification system is supported by both the WHO and NHLBI to promote a consistent nomenclature and classification system.

Pulmonary artery hypertension

Epidemiology of pulmonary hypertension

According to the Centers for Disease Control (CDC), idiopathic pulmonary arterial hypertension (IPAH) is a rare disorder, seen in about one to two persons per million, presenting more frequently in women than men. PH accounted for more than 15,000 deaths and 260,000 hospitalizations

---

* Corresponding author.
E-mail address: bauldoff.1@osu.edu (G.S. Bauldoff).

Box 1. World Health Organization classification nomenclature

Pulmonary arterial hypertension
Idiopathic PAH (formerly primary pulmonary hypertension)
Familial PAH
Associated with:
    Collagen vascular disease
    Congenital systemic to pulmonary shunts (type, dimension,
      correction)
    Portal hypertension
    HIV infection
    Drugs and toxins
    Other (ie, glycogen storage disease, Gaucher disease,
      hereditary hemorrhagic telangiectasia,
      hemoglobinopathies, myeloproliferative disorders,
      splenectomy)
Associated with significant venous or capillary involvement
    Pulmonary veno-occlusive disease
    Pulmonary capillary hemangiomatosis

Pulmonary venous hypertension
Left-sided atrial or ventricular heart disease
Left-sided valvular heart disease

PH associated with hypoxemia
Chronic obstructive pulmonary disease (COPD)
Interstitial lung disease
Alveolar hypoventilation disorders
Chronic exposure to high altitudes

PH caused by chronic thrombotic and embolic disease
Thromboembolic obstruction of proximal pulmonary arteries
Thromboembolic obstruction of distal pulmonary arteries
Pulmonary embolism (tumor, parasites, foreign material)
Miscellaneous (ie, sarcoidosis, histiocytosis X,
    lymphangiomatosis, pulmonary vessel compression from
    adenopathy, tumor or fibrosing mediastinitis).

   Data from Rich S, editor. Primary pulmonary hypertension. Executive Summary from the World Symposium on Primary Pulmonary Hypertension 1998; Evian, France, September 6-10, 1998.

---

in 2002. Of patients hospitalized with PH between 2000 and 2002, women accounted for 61% of the admissions, while 66% were greater than 65 years of age. PH can occur in any population and at any age; however, more women, African-Americans, and the elderly have been hospitalized than any other group. Between 2000 and 2002, 58.3% of deaths related to PH were reported in women as compared with men. Concerns exist that as the population grows older, PH may be more frequently diagnosed [3]. However, the quality of the reported survival data from the CDC is based on *International Classification of Diseases, Ninth Revision* coding, for which there are no comprehensive codes for all causes of PH. Without treatment, survival in severe IPAH has been reported to be less than 3 years [1]. While survival has improved with the development of medical therapies and the advent of lung transplantation, specific data is limited.

Pathophysiology of PAH

The development of PAH is associated with occlusion of the pulmonary arterial tree. The combination of risk factor exposure and susceptible genetic factors can lead to pulmonary vascular bed injury, resulting in increased vasoconstriction. Pulmonary hypertension was formerly believed to be primarily vasconstrictive in etiology, but in the 1990s, vasoprolifera-tive mechanisms were identified. As injury progresses, arterial smooth mus-cle hypertrophies, increased growth is seen in the arterial wall layers, and fibrosis develops in pulmonary arterioles and venules. Development of plex-iform lesions and thrombosis also occurs (Fig. 1) [4].

Risk factors and related conditions to PAH

Exposure to certain risk factors or predisposing conditions may trigger the development of IPAH. Among these, certain anorexigens (appetite

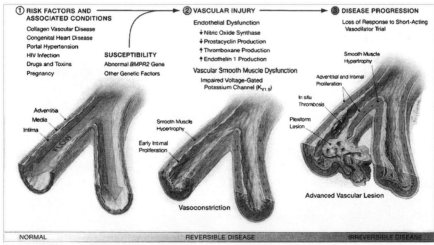

Pulmonary arterial hypertension occurs in susceptible patients as a result of an insult to the pulmonary vascular bed resulting in an injury that progresses to produce the characteristic pathological features. HIV indicates human immunodeficiency virus; *BMPR2*, bone morphogenetic protein receptor II gene.

Fig. 1. Pathophysiology of pulmonary arterial hypertension. *From* Gaine S. Pulmonary hyper-tension. JAMA 2000;284(24):3164; with permission. Copyright © 2000, American Medical Association. All rights reserved.

suppressants) appear to increase the risk for developing PAH (odds ratio or OR 6.3, 95% confidence interval or CI 3.0–13.2) [5]. Stimulants, such as cocaine and amphetamines, have also been associated with IPAH [6,7].

Several systemic illnesses are likewise associated with the development of PAH. Among these are collagen vascular diseases, such as limited sclero-derma, rheumatoid arthritis, and systemic lupus erythematosus (SLE). Additionally, SLE can result in pulmonary vascular bed fibrosis [8]. Con-genital cardiac deformities, which result in chronic shunting of systemic blood to the venous circulation, increase the pressure of the right-sided vas-culature, culminating in damage to the endothelial cells. The subsequent rise in pressure leads to the development of PAH [9]. Portopulmonary hyperten-sion present in advanced liver disease also has been described as resulting in histologic changes in the pulmonary vasculature [10]. HIV infection can be associated with the development of PAH, and evidence implicating the infected T-cells stimulate abnormal vascular endothelial growth [11]. Better survival is seen in those using antiretroviral therapy [12]. The role of herpes virus-8 (Kaposi's sarcoma associated herpes virus) is speculated to play a role in PAH, however evidence is equivocal [13–15].

Genetic influences

Genetic influences have been identified in the development of IPAH and familial PAH. The bone morphogenetic protein receptor, identified in 2000, is part of vascular smooth muscle cell receptors that transform growth fac-tor-β. Mutation of this gene has been identified in 50% of persons with familial PAH and 25% of patients thought to have IPAH. This gene is located at chromosomal region 2q32. Autosomal dominant inheritance with incomplete penetrance is believed to be the mechanism by which this gene is expressed in subsequent generations. With incomplete penetrance, most individuals will not develop the disease but can transmit the mutation to their offspring. Presence of the mutation carries a 10% to 20% risk of developing PAH over the lifetime [16]. Additional mutations or altered func-tion in other genes may be necessary for PAH to develop [17,18]. Another genotype associated with PAH is activin-like kinase type-1, seen in heredi-tary hemorrhagic telangectasia. This receptor is located on endothelial cells that transform growth factor-β and 5-hydroxytryptamine (5-HT or sero-to-nin) transporters. These transformations are associated with pulmonary artery smooth muscle proliferation [19].

Vascular injury and disease progression

Risk factor exposure and susceptibility are the initial insults leading to vascular injury. Such insults lead to endothelial dysfunction. Reduction in nitric oxide synthase, thereby reducing production of nitric oxide and pros-tacyclin, inhibit the potent vasodilator actions of these substances. Throm-boxane production increases, leading to platelet activation and constriction of pulmonary arterioles. Endothelin-1 production also increases, leading to vasoconstriction and promotion of smooth muscle proliferation [4,19].

Smooth muscle dysfunction of the vascular system is also seen. Elevations in plasma serotonin facilitates 5-HT transport into smooth muscle cells, triggering vasoconstriction [16]. Down-regulation of the voltage-gated potassium channel ($K_{v1.5}$) occurs, promoting pulmonary arterial smooth muscle contraction [4,19].

As the disease progresses, additional changes are seen. In situ thrombosis develops. Arterial smooth muscle hypertrophy occurs because of vasoconstriction, and the medial and intimal arterial layers continue to proliferate. Remodeling of the pulmonary vascular system results in plexiform lesions, the most common arteriopathy seen in PAH [20]. Plexiform lesions are comprised of proliferating endothelial cells that arise from monoclonal antibodies. At one time plexiform lesions were thought to be irreversible; however, as understanding of the disease evolves, this may not be the case over the long-term. Plexiform lesions play an important role in increased vascular resistance seen in PAH progression [21].

Pulmonary venous hypertension

Risk factors and cardiovascular diseases related to pulmonary venous hypertension

Pulmonary venous hypertension (PVH) is seen when pulmonary vein outflow is impeded. Disease processes classified under the revised nomenclature and classification system under PVH are left-side atrial (LA) or ventricular (LV) heart disease and left-side valvular heart disease. Left ventricular dysfunction and mitral and aortic valve disease result in increased left atrial pressure, reducing pulmonary vein outflow. Elevated left atrial pressure reflects pulmonary vascular congestion. Other processes that may increase left atrial pressure independent of pulmonary vascular congestion include restrictive cardiomyopathy, myxoma of the left atrium, and constrictive pericarditis [22–24]. None of the Federal Drug Administration (FDA)-approved drugs for PAH have been shown in randomized clinical trials to be beneficial in patients with PVH.

Diastolic heart failure (left ventricular dysfunction with normal ejection fraction) and pulmonary venous hypertension may be bidirectional in disease progression [25]. While PVH passively elevates pulmonary arterial pressure, the development of PH may be related to the endothelial dysfunction seen in severe systolic dysfunction or mitral stenosis [26]. Once remodeling of the pulmonary arteries occurs, the resultant PAH does not respond to reductions in pulmonary venous pressures [27].

Severity of pulmonary hypertension in systolic heart failure (left ventricular dysfunction with reduced ejection fraction) is more commonly related to the severity of diastolic dysfunction than either ejection fraction or cardiac output [23]. Changes of aging such as vascular stiffening, including pulmonary arterial stiffening, appear to be worse in women than in men, leading to increased development of PVH in women [28]. Reduction in atrial compliance and LA pressure increases during systole are reflected by large "V" waves seen in the tracing of the pulmonary arterial waveform [29].

The presence of PH can affect LV diastolic function, modifying LV relaxation and compliance. Above-normal right ventricular (RV) pressure leads to intraventricular septal hypertrophy and influences septal motion, resulting in reduced LV relaxation and compliance. However, RV pressure overload has not been associated with increased LV filling pressure or increases in pulmonary wedge pressure [25].

Mitral stenosis can cause PVH because of increased RV end-diastolic volume and pressure. Pulmonary hypertension detected in the presence of mitral valve disease is an indication for mitral valve surgical intervention [30]. Pulmonary hypertension related to aortic valve stenosis is less common than that experienced with mitral valve stenosis, however between 4% and 29% of persons with severe aortic stenosis are thought to have coexisting PH. The etiology is related to elevations in LV end-diastolic pressure and severe diastolic dysfunction. Without therapy, life expectancy is less than 1.5 years in this population [31].

Other pulmonary hypertension classes

PAH also results from pulmonary embolism and chronic thromboembolic disease. While the right ventricle can sustain output when an acute rise in pulmonary artery pressure (PAP) occurs (up to 50 mm Hg), as the process becomes chronic and PAP rises above 50 mm Hg, RV hypertrophy and RV failure ensue [32]. Hypoxemia is a known pulmonary vasoconstrictor, thus respiratory diseases which culminate in chronic hypoxemia are also associated with the development of PH. Among these are COPD [33], interstitial lung disease, obstructive sleep apnea (especially with obesity hypoventilation) [34], exposure to high altitude, and other causes.

Patient presentation

For patients with PH, nonspecific symptoms are the earliest indication of a problem. Dyspnea on exertion is most common, having been reported in up to 60% of patients [1,35]. Unexplained fatigue and lethargy, especially with activity, is related to the inability to increase cardiac output during periods of increased demand [18]. Initial evaluation often focuses on more common cardiac or pulmonary problems, potentially causing delay in diagnosis. As PH worsens, signs of right ventricular failure emerge, such as peripheral edema and jugular venous distention. With hepatic venous congestion, abdominal pain and anorexia may appear. Later, symptoms include angina and syncope, both reported in up to 40% of PH patients [1]. Syncope can result as a consequence of the inability of the right heart to increase cardiac output with exertion [36].

Diagnosis

History and physical examination

A thorough medical history and comprehensive physical examination are indicated when PH is suspected [35]. Specific assessment to determine the coexistence of medical conditions, such as connective tissue disorders, HIV, sickle cell anemia, liver disease, renal disease, and thromboembolic disease is essential. Inquiry into drug use (legal and illegal), including appetite suppressants and chemotherapeutic agents, is indicated. Family history related to symptoms of PH help to delineate the need for further genetic evaluation [16]. The physical examination should include careful cardiac evaluation. Jugular venous distention indicates an increase in right atrial pressure. With the patient in a 45° semirecumbent position, distention that is seen higher than 9 cm above the sternal angle indicates greater than normal right heart pressure. Pulmonary arterial hypertension can cause jugular venous pulse wave changes that manifest as an increase in the amplitude of both the "a" and "v" waves, with accentuation of the "v" wave being more prominent [37].

Changes in heart sounds also occur. The second heart sound (S2) is increased because of the increased backward pressure against the closing pulmonic valve. During S2, a fixed split between the aortic and pulmonic valve closure sounds may indicate an atrial septal defect. Adventitious heart sounds can also be present in PAH. The third heart sound (S3) can be normal in children and young adults. However, it is abnormal in middle-aged and older adults with PAH because of increased diastolic filling pressure. The S3 can also be present with a reduced LV ejection fraction. The fourth heart sound (S4) can be present in PAH because of a stiffened ventricle. Both the S3 and S4 in PAH are best heard with the patient lying on their left side. Murmurs may also be related to PAH, including those seen with tricuspid regurgitation (holosystolic), pulmonic stenosis or regurgitation (diastolic), or in the presence of a ventricular septal defect [16,37].

Several physical signs present in PAH help determine the underlying cause. Breath sounds, including rales or decreased sounds, are present with pulmonary congestion, but adventitious sounds such as fine rales, wheezing, or prolonged expiration indicate other pulmonary disease. Digital clubbing is most commonly seen in congenital heart disease and is rare in IPAH. Lower extremity edema is often seen in advanced PAH because of right heart failure. As the right heart fails, ascites may develop as a result of elevated vena caval pressure and possible hepatic congestion [16,37].

Diagnostic testing

As part of the comprehensive physical examination, an electrocardio-gram (ECG) and chest x-ray (CXR) should be obtained [35]. The ECG is not sufficiently sensitive to serve as a screening tool in PAH, but can provide evidence of right heart disease and may provide prognostic value. Increase in P-wave amplitude has been linked to increased mortality. When the P wave seen in Lead 2 is greater than or equal to 0.25 millivolts, increased mortality over 6 years has been reported (OR 2.8) while a 1-mm increase in the lead III P wave carries a four- to fivefold increase in mortality [38]. While no correlation has been identified between abnormalities of the CXR and severity of PAH, it may provide information related to enlarged pulmonary arteries and pulmonary arterial pruning, if present. The CXR is also useful for excluding other disease processes that may be responsible for the presenting symptoms [16].

Echocardiography is the noninvasive screening test of choice for pulmo-nary hypertension [16,36]. The test evaluates right and left heart function and size and assesses for congenital deformities. While echocardiography can estimate RV pressure, tricuspid and pulmonic regurgitation jet veloci-ties, as well as PAP, these measures are not always precise [16].

Right heart cardiac catheterization (RHC) is the gold standard for diag-nosis of PAH. Right heart catheterization provides precise pressure mea-surement and is used to determine and monitor therapy. Measurement of the pulmonary capillary wedge pressure during RHC also provides informa-tion regarding pulmonary venous hypertension. Right heart catheterization in patients with suspected PAH carries risk for acute cardiac decompensa-tion, requiring that the physician, nursing and support staff have experience with the procedure. During the procedure, ectopy may occur with catheter manipulation. The development of bradycardia from vagal stimulation can be very problematic, requiring use of atropine to correct the arrhythmia [16,19,39].

Other diagnostic testing

Serologic tests measuring autoantibodies, anticentromere antibodies, and anti-cardiolipin antibodies are appropriate when a connective tissue disorder is suspected from physical examination. HIV testing is appropriate in all per-sons diagnosed with PAH who do not have a clearly identifiable cause. Screening for thyroid disease is recommended, as it may be a risk factor for PAH [16,35]. Ventilation-perfusion scans are indicated to rule out thrombo-embolic disorders. Pulmonary function testing is used to evaluate for pulmo-nary disease with mild abnormalities seen in a majority of PAH patients [18].

Functional capacity evaluation

Exercise testing is an important part of PH evaluation to determine func-tional capacity, maximal activity tolerance, and to determine if other etiologies contribute to the symptomatology. Tests include the 6-minute walk (6MW) and cardiopulmonary exercise testing. Less frequently used tests are exercise echocardiography and exercise RHC. The 6MW tests exercise capacity by asking the patient to walk as fast and as far in 6 minutes as possible; a standardized protocol has been developed [40]. The 6MW predicts survival and is inversely correlated with WHO functional status severity (Box 2) [41]. Paciocco and colleagues [42] reported that for each percent drop in oxygen saturation during the 6MW, there was a 26% increased risk of death. The cardiopulmonary exercise test provides important clinical information beyond the 6MW including peak oxygen consumption (VO_2), work rate, anaerobic threshold, and ventilatory efficiency as determined by dividing minute ventilation by carbon dioxide production during exercise (V_E/VCO_2 slope) [16,35,43]. According to Wensel and colleagues [43], strong predictors of poor PAH survival are low peak VO_2 (risk ratio or RR 0.79, 95% CI 0.705–0.886, $P < .0001$) and low peak systolic blood pressure (RR 0.932, 95% CI 0.906–0.958, $P < .0001$).

Patient management

Treatment depends on the class of pulmonary hypertension (see Box 1). Advanced therapy has been found effective only for PAH (Group 1). As of July 2007, there are six FDA-approved PAH-specific medical therapies. In patients with PVH (Group 2), initial therapy focuses on the treatment of the underlying disease. Montalescot and colleagues [44] reported that the

---

Box 2. World Health Organization functional assessment classification

I. Patients with PH without resulting limitation of physical activity. Ordinary physical activity does not cause undue dyspnea or fatigue, chest pain or near syncope.

II. Patients with PH resulting in slight limitation of physical activity. Asymptomatic at rest. Ordinary physical activity causes dyspnea or fatigue, chest pain or near syncope.

III. Patients with PH resulting in marked limitation of physical activity. Comfortable at rest. Less than ordinary activity causes undue dyspnea or fatigue, chest pain or near syncope.

IV. Patients with PH unable to carry out any physical activity without symptoms. Signs of right-heart failure present. Dyspnea or fatigue may be present at rest. Activity increases discomfort.

Data from Rich S, editor. Primary pulmonary hypertension. Executive Summary from the World Symposium on Primary Pulmonary Hypertension 1998; Evian, France, September 6-10, 1998.

use of prostacyclin in severe LV dysfunction resulted in higher mortality; however, the underlying causes were uncertain. Group 3 PH is related to hypoxemia, and correcting the condition through supplemental oxygen is indicated. Oxygen has been shown to decrease 3-year mortality when used continuously (more than 19 hours per day) as compared with just nocturnal use (22% versus 42%) [45]. Anticoagulation is indicated in PH related to thromboembolic disease (Group 4) and in patients with Class 5 PH, treatment of the underlying cause is indicated.

Medical therapy

Good medical care addresses specific components of PH pathology. Diuretics may be indicated to reduce fluid overload; however, caution with their use is necessary to avoid reducing cardiac output by compromising right ventricular preload. Oxygen therapy is indicated when hypoxemia is noted. Johnson and colleagues [46] reported a survival benefit in a systematic review of anticoagulant use in PAH; however, the survival benefit of anticoagulation has been seen only in IPAH. Digoxin has historically been recommended in those with cardiac impairment caused by PH. Currently, the American Heart Association does not recommend routine use of digoxin in heart failure, as risk may outweigh benefit because of drug sensitivity and high potential for toxicity [47]. Pulmonary rehabilitation (PR) that includes exercise therapy, education, and careful monitoring is a recommended therapy in PH [48]. Research studies testing the use of PR in PH are ongoing. Mereles and colleagues [49] concluded that PR with exercise improved exercise capacity (6MW) at 15 weeks (96 plus or minus 56 m versus 15 plus or minus 54 m in control subjects, $P = .0003$). Improvements were also seen in quality of life, WHO functional class, and workload. Of note, no adverse events were noted throughout the study, as patients were continuously monitored by pulse oximetry and telemetry during exercise.

Advanced therapy

The use of advanced therapy in PH is limited to those with pulmonary arterial hypertension. As the quantity of research related to these therapeutic options has increased, guidelines from the American College of Chest Physicians have been recently updated [50].

Vasoreactivity testing

The use of vasoreactivity testing during right heart catheterization is an important step in determining diagnosis and therapeutic options in PH. A significant response is defined as a reduction in mean PAP of greater than or equal to 10 mm Hg to a value of less than 40 mm Hg [19,51] with normal cardiac output. Only patients with a positive response are considered for calcium channel blocker testing. Common drugs used as the vasodilator in testing include intravenous (IV) epoprostenol, IV adenosine, or inhaled nitric oxide. Nitric oxide is selective for the pulmonary vasculature with a reduced possibility of systemic side effects [52]. Testing is not recommended in patients with severe right heart failure and Class 4 symptoms. Pulmonary hypertension related to collagen vascular disease or portopulmonary syndrome appears to have low vasodilator responsiveness in testing [19,52].

Pharmacologic therapies

Use of calcium channel blockers (CCBs) is limited to patients who demonstrate vasoreactivity and significant improvement in pulmonary arterial pressure while receiving the drug. Sitbon and colleagues [53] reported that of more than 500 participants studied, only 6.8% maintained long-term response to CCB. Specific medications recommended include long-acting nifedipine, diltiazem, or verapamil. However, verapamil may compromise cardiac output because of its negative iontropic properties [50,54]. See Fig. 2 for a pharmacologic decision tree.

Prostanoids include epoprostenol, treprostinil, and iloprost. Endogenous prostacyclin is produced by conversion of arachidonic acid in the vascular endothelium, providing vasodilation and antiplatelet aggregation. Epoprostenol (Flolan, Prostacylin, Prostglandin I2, Prostaglandin X) was the first FDA-approved advanced therapy for PAH. It has a short half-life (less than 6 minutes) and continuous IV infusion via central catheter is required.

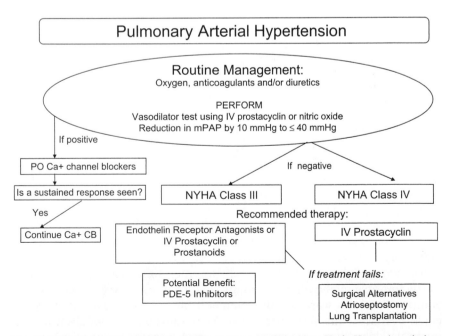

Fig. 2. PAH Treatment Algorithm. *Abbreviations:* NYHA, New York Heart Association; PDE-5, phosphodiesterase type 5.

This is the treatment of choice in severe PAH [51]. In systematic review, IV prostacyclin has been shown to confer benefit in exercise capacity, hemodynamics, and functional performance, and patients with severe PAH appear to have a greater response to epoprostenol [55]. Epoptrostenol carries the burden of continuous infusion, medication storage under refrigeration, and multiple side effects, including jaw pain, myalgia, and diarrhea. Dosage is initiated at 2 ng/kg per minute and increased under strict observation to therapeutic response [56].

Treprostinil (Remodulin) is a prostacyclin analog, administered via subcutaneous or IV infusion. Treprostinil has a half-life of 3 to 4 hours and is stable at room temperature [56]. It has been shown to improve pulmonary hemodynamics and 6MW [57]. Side effects are similar to epoprostenol, with infusion site pain and reaction being the primary limiting factors to continued administration [50,56].

Iloprost (Ventavis) is an inhaled prostacyclin analog administered via a jet nebulizer. Each treatment takes about 15 minutes. The dosage schedule is 6 to 9 times per day, limiting convenience of use [56]. Plasma half-life is 20 to 30 minutes and the most common side effect is cough. Olschewski and colleagues [58] reported increased 6MW distance, improved hemodynamics at 12 weeks, and improvement in functional class symptoms with the use of iloprost. Beraprost is an orally administered prostacyclin analog that is approved only in Japan for use in PAH. The half-life is 35 to 45 minutes following administration. Studies by Galie and colleagues [59] and Barst and colleagues [60] reported improvement in 6MW distance with survival similar to controls.

Endothelin-1 is a potent vasoconstrictor overexpressed in PAH [61]. Two different receptors (A and B) have been identified for endothelin in pulmonary vascular smooth muscle. Stimulation of the endothelin-A receptor causes vasoconstriction and smooth muscle growth. Endothelin-B receptors are located both in endothelial cells and smooth muscle cells and receptor response is dependent on their location. Stimulation of endothelin-B receptors located on endothelial cells results in release of prostacyclin and nitric oxide. However, when endothelin-B receptors located in smooth muscle are stimulated, vasoconstriction and smooth muscle growth occur [62].

Endothelin receptor antagonists (ERA) are a class of drugs that block stimulation of the endothelin receptors in PAH. Endothelin receptor antagonists improve exercise capacity and functional class, reduce dyspnea, and alter hemodynamics, including mean PAP, PVR, and cardiac index [50,63]. Bosentan (Tracleer) is a nonselective ERA that is administered orally. Rubin and colleagues reported that bosentan improved 6MW distance, dyspnea, and functional class at 16 weeks [62]. Bosentan has been shown to significantly improve quality of life in idiopathic PAH and PAH associated with connective tissue disease [64]. Bosentan half-life is 5 hours and side effects include headache and nasopharyngitis. Hepatotoxicity should be carefully monitored [56]. Sitaxsentan is an endothelin-A receptor-specific ERA, which is approved for use in Canada and parts of Europe. Improvements in exercise capacity, functional class, and hemodynamics have been reported with its use in randomized clinical trials [50,51]. Ambrisentan, (Letairis) an endothelin-A specific ERA, has shown positive effect on functional capacity [65] and this drug received FDA approval June, 2007 [66]. Ambrisentan requires monthly laboratory testing similar to bosentan. Additional clinical drug trials continue for ambristentan [50].

Phosphodiesterase 5 (PDE5) inhibitors stimulate relaxation of pulmonary vascular smooth muscle. The mechanism of action increases availability of cyclic guanosine nonophosphate, a potent pulmonary vasodilator [50]. Sildenafil (Revatio) is a specific PDE5 inhibitor. Originally approved for use with erectile dysfunction, it is now approved for use in PAH. The half-life is 4 hours, with major side effects including headache, stomach upset, and flushing [56]. This drug improves functional capacity, functional class, and hemodynamics [67]. When compared with ERAs, sildenafil, when added to conventional therapy, has resulted in RV mass reduction [68].

Other therapeutic options, such as nitric oxide or arginine supplementation, do not have sufficient evidence to support or refute their use. Rigorous randomized clinical trials are recommended in the current clinical guidelines [51]. Combination therapy that includes prostanoids, ERAs, and PDE5 inhibitors is currently under investigation [50,69]. Ghofrani and colleagues [70] reported greater reductions in PVR and PAP with combined sildenafil and inhaled iloprost.

Surgical therapy
Lung transplantation. In the late 1980s and through the mid-1990s, lung transplantation (LT) was considered the mainstay of therapy for advanced PH. However, with the advent of epoprostenol and other medical therapies, the need for LT has been significantly curtailed. In 1996, the percentage of lung transplants performed for PH was 5.4% (43 of 791) as compared with only 2.9% (41 of 1,407) in 2005 [71]. While LT remains a viable treatment for advanced PH, it is usually not employed until there has been a demonstrated failure of medical therapy. The need for chronic immunosuppressive medications, the risk of opportunistic infections and graft rejection, along with less than ideal 5-year survival rates following LT, are all reasons for delaying this therapy as long as possible. However, when necessary, LT can significantly enhance the life of the patient with PH.

The time to offer LT to the patient with PH depends on the severity of their disease and the early response to medications. Transplantation should not be offered too early because of the aforementioned risks. Conversely, referring patients too late can result in insufficient time to receive a transplant. Because of the relative scarcity of donor organs, once the patient is listed, the average waiting time for an organ can exceed 2 years. With the new lung allocation system, wait time is based on multiple factors, modifying wait times according to the patient's condition. Therefore, it is critical to continually evaluate the patient with PH and refer them for LT when appropriate. Recently, a panel of experts made recommendations for when patients with PH should be referred for LT [72]. Patients who present with NYHA functional class III and IV should be referred for LT while being started on medical therapy. If medical therapy is successful, then the patient can be removed from the transplant list, while those patients whose disease progresses should proceed on to transplantation. Many times the progression of functional decline will slow with medical therapy, yet inexorably continue. In these cases, epoprostenol and other medications may extend the time necessary to secure transplantable organs by "bridging" the patient to LT [73]. Additionally, the WHO has compiled a list of those indicators that herald poor outcomes to assist health care providers in the proper timing of transplant referral (Box 3) [74].

The type of transplant procedure offered to patients with PH has been debated and depends upon the experience of the individual transplant center, the projected waiting time at a given center, and the etiology of the PH. Combined heart-lung transplant (HLT) was the initial procedure performed in the 1980s, but this has now given way to the more popular bilateral lung transplant (BLT) procedure. Bilateral lung transplant allows for complete replacement of the diseased pulmonary vascular bed, and experience has shown that even in cases of severe right ventricular dysfunction resulting from the PH, this dysfunction will often return to normal obviating the need for replacement of the heart [75]. Today, HLT is generally reserved for PH resulting from Eisenmenger's physiology, where the coexisting heart defect is too complex to repair surgically. If projected waiting times for two lung grafts is anticipated to be long or the patient's condition is deteriorating, some centers will offer single lung transplant (SLT) for PH.

Following LT for any reason, the early mortality (within the first 30 days) can be a result of primary graft failure (30.5%), infection (23.5%), cardiovascular complications (11.5%), technical factors (8.3%), acute graft

---

Box 3. WHO indications for lung transplantation in pulmonary arterial hypertension

Failure of medical therapy in the setting of:
New York Heart Association functional class III or IV (should refer for transplant evaluation while assessing response to initial medical therapy)
Mean right atrial pressure ≥ 10 mm Hg
Mean pulmonary arterial pressure ≥ 50 mm Hg
Cardiac index ≤ 2.0 L per min/m²

Data from Rich S, editor. Primary pulmonary hypertension. Executive Summary from the World Symposium on Primary Pulmonary Hypertension 1998; Evian, France, September 6-10, 1998.

rejection (4.9%), and bronchiolitis (0.5%) [76]. In addition to these risks assumed by all LT recipients, following transplantation the survival of the recipient with PH may be determined by additional factors. Among these is the degree of PH present before the procedure. Doyle and colleagues [72] reported that analysis of the International Society of Heart and Lung Transplantation Registry for those patients transplanted between 1995 and 1997 suggested that those recipients with a pretransplant pulmonary arterial systolic pressure of greater than 40 mm Hg were associated with an increased 5-year posttransplant mortality. In addition, the type of graft received may impact survival. Recipients who have received an SLT tend to have a higher degree of reperfusion lung injury that can severely complicate the immediate postoperative course [77]. A survival advantage of BLT, compared with SLT, in idiopathic PAH has been reported, but one study has suggested that this may only be true for recipients with high preoperative PAP (greater than 40 mm Hg) [78,79]. While hemodynamics improved following both BLT and HLT procedures, studies have shown superior hemodynamics and cardiac outputs in those receiving heart-lung grafts [80]. Despite this, the survival benefit of HLT over either SLT or BLT has not been demonstrated in most series [81,82]. Overall, 1-year survival for PH patients receiving LT is somewhat less than those patients afflicted with other disorders, and currently stands at 72%, while 5-year survival approaches 40% [83].

Atrial septostomy. Atrial septostomy is another surgical option that results in the surgical creation of an atrial septal defect. The atrial septum is punctured and the resulting ostomy is dilated with a balloon until optimum size is achieved. The procedure is not commonly used, especially with the advent of advanced therapy and lung transplantation. It remains a therapeutic option for patients with right heart failure who have been maximized on medical therapy [84]. It is contraindicated in patients with significantly elevated PVR, low oxygen saturation, or severe right heart failure caused by the potential for substantial right-to-left shunting that may reduce pulmonary blood flow [72]. A recent study reported that balloon atrial septostomy improved cardiac index and functional class with no significant complications related to the procedure [85].

Nursing implications

Nursing plays a central role in the management, education, and support of persons with PH. Receiving a diagnosis of pulmonary hypertension can be devastating to the patient and their family. The patient, when presenting with nebulous symptoms such as fatigue and dyspnea with exertion, does not expect to receive a life-threatening diagnosis.

Nursing in PH takes place across the therapeutic milieu spectrum, from primary outpatient care through critical care management and across the lifespan. Individualized nursing care specific to the patient's condition, comorbidities, and therapeutic plan should be implemented. The patient's social situation and support network should be evaluated. A holistic review of the patient's circumstances will allow the nurse to proactively identify and address potential problems that could reduce the patient's participation in their treatment plan or in the effectiveness of their therapy.

Nurses are vital in the management of the PH patient with advanced therapy. Crucial activities include initiation of therapy and therapy continuation. As part of a collaborative interdisciplinary health care team, nurses serve as the primary interface with the patient and their family. Advanced assessment skills of nurses provide important early evaluation for therapy response and progression of illness. Goal setting with the patient and family promotes concordance with the treatment plan.

Patient education is paramount in PH. Teaching about the underlying pathophysiologic processes gives foundation to all other patient education. Education should include recognition of and response to symptoms, activity limitations, and therapeutic alternatives from medications through surgical treatments. Burdensome therapeutic regimens risk the potential for poor adherence. Nurses have the unique role of translating complex therapy into specific actions in day-to-day life, resulting in a realistic and practical treatment plan. Diagnostic testing should be described in language appropriate for the patient, including what they will experience, how long the test takes, potential complications, and so forth.

Identification and referral to relevant community resources is essential. All patients with pulmonary hypertension should be referred to the Pulmonary Hypertension Association (PHA) (www.phassociation.org). This nonprofit organization provides support, education, advocacy, and awareness for persons with pulmonary hypertension. The PHA has both patient and medical professional components for access to up-to-date information. The organization convenes a biennial conference for patients and health care professionals. While the PHA headquarters in the United States, it provides services to persons with PH throughout the world.

References

[1] Rich S, Dantzker DR, Ayres SM, et al. Primary pulmonary hypertension: a national prospective study. Ann Intern Med 1987;107(2):216–23.
[2] Rubin J. Introduction: diagnosis and management of pulmonary arterial hypertension: ACCP evidence-based clinical guidelines. Chest 2004;126(Suppl 1):7S–10S.
[3] Hyduk A, Croft JB, Ayala C, et al. Pulmonary hypertension surveillance United States 1980–2002. Morbidity and Mortality Weekly Report 2005;54(SS05):1–28.
[4] Gaine S. Pulmonary hypertension. JAMA 2000;284(24):3160–8.
[5] Abenhaim L, Moride Y, Brenot F, et al. Appetite-suppressant drugs and risk of primary pulmonary hypertension. N Engl J Med 2001;335(9):609–16.
[6] Schaiberger PH, Kennedy TC, Miller FC, et al. Pulmonary hypertension associated with long-term inhalation of "crack" methamphetamine. Chest 1993;104:614–6.

[7] Albertson TE, Walby EF, Derlet RW. Stimulant-induced pulmonary toxicity. Chest 1995; 108(4):1140–9.

[8] Gurubhagavatula I, Palevsky HI. Pulmonary hypertension in systemic autoimmune disease. Rheumatic Disease Clinics of North America 1997;23(2):365–94.

[9] Grossman W, Braunwald E. Pulmonary hypertension. In: Braunwald E, editor. Heart disease: a textbook of cardiovascular medicine. 4th edition. Philadelphia: Saunders; 1992. p. 786–882.

[10] Mandell MS, Groves BM. Pulmonary hypertension in chronic liver disease. Clin Chest Med 1996;17:17–33.

[11] Ascherl G, Hohenadl C, Schatz O, et al. Infection with human immunodeficiency syndrome-associated vasculopathy. Blood 1999;93(12):4232–41.

[12] Mehta NJ, Khan IA, Mehta RN, et al. HIV-related pulmonary hypertension. Chest 2000; 118(4):1133–41.

[13] Cool CD, Rai PR, Yeager ME, et al. Expression of human herpes virus 8 in primary pulmonary hypertension. N Engl J Med 2003;349(12):1113–22.

[14] Laney AS, DeMarco T, Peters JS, et al. Kaposi sarcoma-associated herpes virus and primary and secondary pulmonary hypertension. Chest 2005;127(3):762–7.

[15] Henke-Gendo C, Mengel M, Hoeper MM, et al. Absence of Kaposi's sarcoma-associated herpes virus in patients with pulmonary arterial hypertension. Am J Respir Crit Care Med 2005;172(12):1581–5.

[16] McGoon M, Gutterman D, Steen V, et al. Screen, early detection and diagnosis of pulmonary arterial hypertension. ACCP evidence-based clinical practice guidelines. Chest 2004; 126(1):14S–34S.

[17] Machado RD, James V, Southwood M, et al. Investigation of second genetic hits at the BMPR2 locus as a modulator of disease progression in familial pulmonary arterial hypertension. Circulation 2005;111(5):607–13.

[18] Rubin LJ. Pulmonary arterial hypertension. Proc Am Thorac Soc 2006;3:111–5.

[19] McLaughlin VV, McGoon MD. Pulmonary arterial hypertension. Circulation 2006;114(13): 1417–31.

[20] Rubin LJ. Pathology and pathophysiology of primary pulmonary hypertension. Am J Cardiol 1995;75:51A–4A.

[21] Ghamra ZW, Dweik RA. Primary pulmonary hypertension: an overview of epidemiology and pathogenesis. Cleve Clin J Med 2003;70(Suppl 1):S2–8.

[22] Abramson SV, Burke JF, Kelly JJ, et al. Pulmonary hypertension predicts mortality and morbidity in patients with dilated cardiomyopathy. Ann Intern Med 1992;116(11):888–95.

[23] Enriquez-Sarano M, Rossi A, Seward JB, et al. Determinants of pulmonary hypertension in left ventricular dysfunction. J Am Coll Cardiol 1997;29(1):153–9.

[24] Alexopoulos D, Lazzam C, Borrico S, et al. Isolated chronic mitral regurgitation with preserved systolic left ventricular function and severe pulmonary hypertension. J Am Coll Cardiol 1989;14(2):319–22.

[25] Shapiro BP, Nishimura RA, McGoon MD, et al. Diagnostic dilemmas: diastolic heart failure caused pulmonary hypertension and pulmonary hypertension causing diastolic dysfunction. Advances in Pulmonary Hypertension 2006;5(1):13–20.

[26] Moraes DL, Colucci WS, Givertz MM. Secondary pulmonary hypertension in chronic heart failure: the role of the endothelium in pathophysiology and management. Circulation 2000; 102(14):1718–23.

[27] Delgado JF, Conde E, Sanchez V, et al. Pulmonary vascular remodeling in pulmonary hypertension due to chronic heart failure. Eur J Heart Fail 2005;7(6):1011–6.

[28] Redfield MM, Jacobsen SJ, Bourlaug BA, et al. Age- and gender-related ventricular-vascular stiffening: a community based study. Circulation 2005;112(15):2254–62.

[29] Pichard AD, Diaz R, Marchant E, et al. Large V waves in the pulmonary capillary wedge pressure tracing with mitral valve regurgitation: the influence of the pressure/volume relationship of the V wave size. Clin Cardiol 1983;6:534–41.

[30] Bonow RO, Carbello B, Kanu C, et al. ACCC/AHA guidelines for the management of patients with valvular heart disease: a report of the American College of Cardiology/American Heart Association task force on practice guidelines (writing committee to revise the 1998 guidelines for the management of patients with valvular heart disease). Circulation 2006; 114(5):384–431.

[31] Silver K, Aurigemma G, Krendel S, et al. Pulmonary artery hypertension in severe aortic stenosis: incidence and mechanism. Am Heart J 1993;125:146–50.

[32] Moser KM, Auger WR, Fedullo PF. Chronic major-vessel thromboembolic pulmonary hypertension. Circulation 1990;81(6):1735–43.

[33] Barbera JA, Peinado VI, Santos S. Pulmonary hypertension in chronic obstructive pulmonary disease. Eur Respir J 2003;21(5):892–905.

[34] Bady E, Achkar A, Pascal S, et al. Pulmonary arterial hypertension in patients with sleep aponea syndrome. Thorax 2000;55(11):934–9.

[35] Barst RJ, McGoon M, Torbicki A, et al. Diagnosis and differential assessment of pulmonary arterial hypertension. J Am Coll Cardiol 2004;43(12 Suppl S):40S–7S.

[36] Mesquita SM, Castro CRP, Ikari NM, et al. Likelihood of left main coronary artery compression based on pulmonary truck diameter in patients with pulmonary hypertension. Am J Med 2004;116:369–75.

[37] Bull TM. Physical examination in pulmonary arterial hypertension. Adv Pulm Hyperten 2005;4(3):6–10.

[38] Bossone E, Paciocco G, Iarussi D, et al. The prognostic value of the ECG in primary pulmonary hypertension. Chest 2002;121(2):513–8.

[39] Oudiz RJ, Langleben D. Cardiac catheterization in pulmonary arterial hypertension: an updated guide to proper use. Adv Pulm Hyperten 2005;4(3):15–25.

[40] Crapo RO, Casaburi R, Coates AL, et al. ATS Statement: guidelines for the six-minute walk test. Am J Respir Crit Care Med 2002;166(1):111–7.

[41] Guyatt GH, Sullivan MJ, Thompson PJ, et al. The 6-minute walk: a new measure of exercise capacity in patients with chronic heart failure. Can Med Assoc J 1985;132(8):919–23.

[42] Paciocco G, Martinez FJ, Bossone E, et al. Oxygen desaturation on the six-minute walk test and mortality in untreated primary pulmonary hypertension. Eur Respir J 2001;17(4):647–52.

[43] Wensel R, Opitz CF, Anker SD, et al. Assessment of survival in patients with primary pulmonary hypertension. Importance of cardiopulmonary exercise testing. Circulation 2002; 106:319–24.

[44] Montalescot G, Drobinski G, Meurin R, et al. Effects of prostacyclin on the pulmonary vascular tone and cardiac contractility of patients with pulmonary hypertension secondary of end-stage heart failure. Am J Cardiol 1998;82:749–55.

[45] Nocturnal Oxygen Therapy Trial Group. Continuous or nocturnal oxygen therapy in hypoxemic chronic obstructive pulmonary disease: a clinical trial. Ann Intern Med 1980;93(3): 391–8.

[46] Johnson SR, Mehta S, Granton JT. Anticoagulation in pulmonary arterial hypertension: a qualitative systematic review. Eur Respir J 2006;28:999–1012.

[47] Hunt SA, Baker DW, Chin MH, et al. ACC/AHA guidelines for the evaluation and management of chronic heart failure in the adult: executive summary. A report of the American College of Cardiology/American Heart Association task force on practice guidelines. J Am Coll Cardiol 2001;38(7):2101–13.

[48] Ries AL, Bauldoff GS, Carlin BW, et al. Pulmonary rehabilitation. Joint ACCP/AACVPR evidence-based clinical practice guidelines. Chest 2007;131(Suppl 5):4S–42S.

[49] Mereles D, Ehlken N, Kreuscher S, et al. Exercise and respiratory training improve exercise capacity and quality of life in patients with severe chronic pulmonary hypertension. Circulation 2006;114:1482–9.

[50] Badesch DB, Abman SH, Simonneau G, et al. Medical therapy for pulmonary arterial hypertension. Updated ACCP evidence-based clinical practice guidelines. Chest 2007; 131(6):1917–28.

[51] Badesch DB, Abman SH, Ahearn GS, et al. Medical therapy for pulmonary arterial hypertension. ACCP evidence-based clinical practice guidelines. Chest 2004;126(Suppl 1): 35S–62S.

[52] Morales-Blanhir J, Santos S, de Jover L, et al. Clinical value of vasodilator test with inhaled nitric oxide for predicting long-term response to oral vasodilators in pulmonary hypertension. Respir Med 2004;98:225–34.

[53] Sitbon O, Humbert M, Jais X, et al. Long-term response to calcium channel blockers in idiopathic pulmonary arterial hypertension. Circulation 2005;111:3105–11.

[54] Beutz MA, Bull TM, Badesch DB. Oral therapies for PAH: State-of-the-art and investigational approaches. Adv Pulm Hyperten 2006;5(4):13–7.

[55] Paramothayan NS, Lasserson TJ, Wells AU, et al. Prostacyclin for pulmonary hypertension in adults (Review). Cochrane Database Syst Rev 2005;2:1–61, CD002994.

[56] Deglin JP, Vallerand AP. Davis drug guide. Philadelphia: F.A. Davis Co.; 2006.

[57] Simonneau G, Barst RJ, Galie N, et al. Continuous subcutaneous infusion of treprostinil, a prostacyclin analogue, in patients with pulmonary arterial hypertension: a double-blind, randomized, placebo-controlled trial. Am J Respir Crit Care Med 2002;165:800–4.

[58] Olschewski H, Simonneau G, Galie N, et al. Inhaled iloprost for severe pulmonary hypertension. N Engl J Med 2002;347(5):322–9.

[59] Galie N, Humbert M, Vachiery JL, et al. Effects of beraprost sodium, an oral prostacyclin analogue, in patients with pulmonary arterial hypertension: a randomized, double-blind, placebo-controlled trial. J Am Coll Cardiol 2002;39:1496–502.

[60] Barst RJ, McGoon M, McLaughlin V, et al. Beraprost therapy for pulmonary arterial hypertension. J Am Coll Cardiol 2003;41:2119–25.

[61] Giaid A, Yangisawa M, Langleben D, et al. Expression of endothelin-1 in the lungs of patients with pulmonary hypertension. N Engl J Med 1993;328:1732–9.

[62] Rubin LJ, Badesch DB, Barst RJ, et al. Bosentan therapy for pulmonary arterial hypertension. N Engl J Med 2002;346:896–903.

[63] Liu C, Chen J. Endothelin receptor antagonists for pulmonary arterial hypertension (Review). Cochrane Database Syst Rev 2006;3:1–22, CD004434.

[64] Keogh AM, McNeil KD, Wlodarczyk J, et al. Quality of life in pulmonary arterial hypertension: improvement and maintenance with bostentan. J Heart Lung Transplant 2007;26(2): 181–7.

[65] Galie N, Badesch D, Oudiz R, et al. Ambristentan therapy for pulmonary arterial hypertension. J Am Coll Cardiol 2005;46:529–35.

[66] Federal Drug Administration. FDA News. 2007. Available at: http://www.fda.gov/bbs/topics/NEWS/2007/NEW01653.html. Accessed July 11, 2007.

[67] Galie N, Ghofrani HA, Torbicki A, et al. Sildenafil citrate therapy for pulmonary arterial hypertension. N Engl J Med 2005;353:2148–57.

[68] Wilkins MR, Paul GA, Strange JW, et al. Sildenafil versus endothelin receptor antagonist for pulmonary hypertension (SERAPH) study. Am J Respir Crit Care Med 2005;171:1292–7.

[69] Benza RL, Park MH, Keogh A, et al. Management of pulmonary arterial hypertension with a focus on combination therapies. J Heart Lung Transplant 2007;26(5):437–46.

[70] Ghofrani HA, Wiedemann R, Rose F, et al. Combination therapy with oral sildenafil and inhaled iloprost for severe pulmonary hypertension. Ann Intern Med 2002;136:515–22.

[71] Department of Health and Human Services, Health Resources and Services Administration. 2006 Annual report of the U.S. organ procurement and transplantation network and the scientific registry of transplant recipients: transplant data 1996–2005. Healthcare systems bureau, division of transplantation, Rockville, MD; United Network for Organ Sharing. Richmond (VA); University Renal Research and Education Association. Ann Arbor, MI.

[72] Doyle RL, McCrory D, Channick RN, et al. Surgical treatments/interventions for pulmonary arterial hypertension: ACCP evidence-based clinical practice guidelines. Chest 2004; 126(Suppl 1):63S–71S.

[73] Conte JV, Gaine SP, Orens JB, et al. The influence of continuous intravenous prostacyclin therapy for primary pulmonary hypertension on the timing and outcome of transplantation. J Heart Lung Transplant 1998;17(7):679–85.

[74] Rich S, editor. Executive summary from the World Symposium on Primary Pulmonary Hypertension 1998. Evian (France). 1998. Cosponsored by the World Health Organization. Accessed April 14, 2000, from the World Wide Web, Available at: http://www.who.int/ncd/cvd/pph.html.

[75] Pasque MK, Trulock EP, Cooper JD, et al. Single lung transplantation for pulmonary hypertension. Single institution experience in 34 patients. Circulation 1995;92(8):2252–8.

[76] Trulock EP, Edwards LB, Taylor DO, et al. The registry of the international society of heart and lung transplantation: twentieth official adult lung and heart-lung transplant report—2003. J Heart Lung Transplant 2003;22(6):625–35.

[77] Boujoukos AJ, Martich GD, Vega JD, et al. Reperfusion injury in single lung transplant recipients with pulmonary hypertension and emphysema. J Heart Lung Transplant 1997;16:440–8.

[78] Chapelier A, Vouhe P, Macchiarini P, et al. Comparative outcome of heart-lung and lung transplantation for pulmonary hypertension. J Thorac Cardiovasc Surg 1993;106:229–307.

[79] Conte JV, Borja MJ, Patel CB, et al. Lung transplantation for primary and secondary pulmonary hypertension. Ann Thorac Surg 2001;72:1673–80.

[80] Sandoval J, Gaspar J, Pulido T, et al. Graded balloon dilation atrial septostomy in severe primary pulmonary hypertension: a therapeutic alternative for patients nonresponsive to vasodilator treatment. J Am Coll Cardiol 1998;32:297–304.

[81] Ueno T, Smith JA, Snell GI, et al. Bilateral sequential single lung transplantation for pulmonary hypertension and Eisenmenger's syndrome. Ann Thorac Surg 2000;2:381–7.

[82] Mendeloff EN, Meyers BF, Sundt TM, et al. Lung transplantation for pulmonary vascular disease. Ann Thorac Surg 2002;73:209–19.

[83] US Department of Health and Human Resources. 2003. Annual report of the US scientific registry for transplant recipients and the organ procurement and transplantation network: transplant data 1989–2001. 2003. Rockville (MD), UNOS, Richmond, VA.

[84] Olsson JK, Zamanian RT, Feinstein JA, et al. Surgical and interventional therapies for pulmonary arterial hypertension. Semin Respir Crit Care Med 2005;26(4):417–28.

[85] Kurzyna M, Dabrowski M, Bielecki D, et al. Atrial septostomy in treatment of end-stage right heart failure in patients with pulmonary hypertension. Chest 2007;131(4):977–83.

NURSING CLINICS
OF NORTH AMERICA

Nurs Clin N Am 43 (2008) 37–53

ELSEVIER
SAUNDERS

Risk Profile for Cardiovascular Morbidity and Mortality After Lung Transplantation

Annette De Vito Dabbs, RN, PhD[a],*, Mi-Kyung Song, RN, PhD[b]

[a]Department of Acute & Tertiary Care, School of Nursing, University of Pittsburgh, Pittsburgh, 3500 Victoria Street, Pittsburgh, PA 15261, USA
[b]Adult/Geriatric Health Division, School of Nursing, University of North Carolina, 433 Carrington Hall, CB#7640, Chapel Hill, NC 27599-7460, USA

The number of persons undergoing lung transplantation has steadily increased with notable improvements in graft and recipient survival. Currently, survival rates at 1 and 3 years post–lung transplant are 84% and 62%, largely because of the availability of more effective pharmacological agents to treat infection and rejection, but survival rates still lag considerably behind those of other sold organ transplants [1].

Rejection of the allograft, the body's normal immune response to foreign antigens, occurs more frequently and has a propensity to recur in lung recipients compared with recipients of other organs [2,3]. In an attempt to combat the increased susceptibility to rejection, the immunosuppression regimen after lung transplantation is more intense than regimens for other organ recipients. The maintenance regimen for approximately 75% of lung recipients is composed of a calcineurin inhibitor, either tacrolimus or cyclosporine, plus a purine synthesis antagonist, and prednisone, but no specific combination predominates [4]. While immunosuppression has significantly contributed to the success of lung transplantation, it is increasingly implicated in poor long-term cardiovascular outcomes. Untoward effects of the immunosuppressive agents include the development or exacerbation of comorbidities, such as diabetes, hypertension, and hyperlipidemia, which complicate the medical management of lung recipients, increase their risk

The work was supported by K01NR9385, National Institute of Nursing Research (PI, A. De Vito Dabbs).

* Corresponding author.
  E-mail address: ajdst42@pitt.edu (A. De Vito Dabbs).

of subsequent cardiovascular adverse events, and jeopardize their long-term survival [5].

Of the nearly 10,000 individuals who received a lung transplant between 1998 and 2003, 60% required treatment for new-onset hypertension, 32% for diabetes, and 20% for hyperlipidemia by the end of year 1 [6], and these proportions increased considerably for 5-year survivors [4]. Unfortunately, the prevalence of these comorbid conditions is increasing because of the availability of newer and more potent immunosuppressive agents, together with the rise in comorbidities that accompanies the increasing age of acceptable transplant candidates and surviving recipients [7]. Rates are likely to increase further because recent guidelines put forth by expert panels on the detection, evaluation, and treatment of diabetes [8,9], hypertension [10], and high blood cholesterol [11] recommend lower diagnostic thresholds for high-risk populations including solid organ transplant recipients on chronic immunosuppression.

Each of these comorbid conditions is an independent risk factor for the development of subsequent cardiovascular events. Consequently, the absolute death rate from cardiovascular disease in all transplant recipients is twice the rate in the general population. In fact, cardiovascular disease is the primary cause of death after heart [12] and kidney transplantation [13], and among the three most common causes of death after liver transplantation [14,15]. Cardiovascular morbidity currently accounts for approximately 10% of deaths after lung transplantation [12,16]. The cardiovascular mortality rate is lower among lung recipients because the length of survival is lower after lung transplantation compared with heart, kidney, and liver. However, the risk factors that contribute to cardiovascular morbidity and mortality develop earlier, more frequently, and more often in combination after lung transplant compared with other solid organ transplants. With the use of aggressive preoperative cardiac interventions, cardiovascular disease is no longer an absolute contraindication for lung transplantation [17]. As survival after lung transplantation nears that of other solid organ recipients, the incidence of cardiovascular morbidity and mortality is expected to rise. Therefore, the prevention and management of immunosuppressant-induced cardiovascular complications becomes paramount for achieving long-term success after lung transplantation.

Prevalence and risk factors for comorbidities

Diabetes

New-onset diabetes, one of the first conditions to be recognized as a complication after organ transplantation, is associated with poor recipient and graft survival [18,19]. The evidence linking glucose intolerance after transplant to immunosuppressive agents is unequivocal, although different agents vary in the extent to which they induce diabetes [20]. Estimations of the adverse effects associated with the most common immunosuppressive agents are presented in Table 1 [21–23]. The association between corticosteroid use and diabetes is reportedly as high as 46% and the diabetogenic effects appear to be dose-related [24]. The use of steroid-free immunosuppression protocols after other solid organ transplants, including kidney and liver, have virtually eliminated the development of posttransplant diabetes, but withdrawal of prednisone in lung recipients has not been successful in preventing rejection, and is therefore not an option for reducing diabetes after lung transplant [25].

The onset of diabetes mellitus can be insidious and recipients may experience glucose intolerance yet be asymptomatic [26]. Recipients are initially at greatest risk for developing diabetes during the first 6 months after transplant, but the number increases linearly and progressively thereafter, with new-onset diabetes developing in some recipients up to 15 years after transplantation [27,28]. Posttransplant diabetes is not always permanent; it may normalize, remit, or recur several years after transplantation. Chronic hyperglycemia associated with diabetes carries long-term risks for microvascular and macrovascular adverse events, thereby increasing cardiovascular morbidity and mortality [29,30]. In fact, cardiovascular events are listed as the primary cause of death in about 65% of transplant recipients with diabetes [31].

Hypertension

Posttransplant hypertension appears to be a major risk factor determining graft and patient survival [21]. Over 60% of lung transplant recipients with previously normal blood pressure develop hypertension by the end of the first year posttransplant; prevalence increases to 75% in 7-year survivors [32]. These recipients require antihypertensive therapies, usually with more than one agent to achieve control [33]. The mechanisms for hypertension after transplant include vasoconstriction, long-term vascular structural changes, and relative salt and water retention caused by the calcineurin inhibitors and corticosteroids [34]. Nocturnal hypertension with a high night-to-day ratio, the reverse of the normal diurnal blood pressure rhythm, has also been documented in transplant recipients [35], Although the mechanism is unknown, this phenomenon is associated with adverse cardiovascular outcomes.

Table 1
Estimation of adverse effects for common immunosuppressive agents [21,22]

	Diabetogenicity	Hypertension	Dyslipidemia
Cyclosporine	++	++	++
Tacrolimus	++	+	+
Sirolimus	none	none	+++
Prednisone	+++	++	++

+ signs indicate the degree of likelihood that each medication will cause the adverse effect, the more + signs the greater the likelihood.

Hyperlipidemia

Transplant recipients have a high incidence of abnormalities in lipid metabolism, including hypercholesterolemia and hypertriglyceridemia [36]. Hyperlipidemia is common after lung transplantation, affecting 20% of lung recipients in year 1 and rising to nearly 50% in 5-year survivors [4]. As in the general population, this condition is a risk factor for cardiovascular disease, and after transplant is also associated with a poorer prognosis for graft survival [37,38]. The type of immunosuppressant regimen appears to influence the frequency of this abnormality after transplantation; many of the immunosuppressants, particularly prednisone, sirolimus, and cyclosporine, are associated with increased levels of serum lipids [36]. The use of tacrolimus tends to be associated with better serum lipid profiles than those seen with cyclosporine-based regimens [37–39], and change from cyclosporine to tacrolimus is generally associated with improved lipid profiles. Several studies using preventive lipid-lowering HMG-CoA reductase inhibitors (statins) show promise in modulating the development and progression of atherosclerosis and improving graft function and survival after lung transplantation [40–42].

Concomitant comorbidities

Diabetes, hypertension, and hyperlipidemia are serious complications that adversely affect survival, long-term viability of the lung allograft, and quality of life. Furthermore, lung recipients are likely to develop multiple comorbid conditions over their lifetime. By 3 years after lung transplant, 90% of recipients developed at least one of these three comorbid conditions and 60% developed at least two of the three comorbid conditions [43]. The impact of co-occurring comorbidities after lung transplantation has not been explored, however evidence from the general population and other solid organ transplant recipients demonstrates that effects are additive with regard to risk for subsequent cardiovascular events.

Transplant recipients with diabetes have an increased incidence of coexisting conditions, particularly dyslipidemia and hypertension, which contribute to higher risk for cardiovascular morbidity and mortality [26,44]. The coexistence of hypertension and diabetes is particularly ominous because of the strong linkages of both conditions with cardiovascular adverse events [45,46]. Glucose intolerance or hypertension in the presence of hyperlipidemia after transplantation confers a higher risk of new cardiovascular heart disease within 5 years [11].

The so-called "metabolic syndrome," a constellation of concomitant cardiovascular risk factors [11], has an estimated prevalence of 23.7% in US adults [47], and is highly age dependent, rising to more than 40% in Americans older than 60. Metabolic syndrome is determined by the presence of three or more of the following: hypertension (systolic blood pressure [SBP] $\geq$ 130, diastolic blood pressure [DBP] $\geq$ 85), truncal obesity (waist circumference > 88 cm for women, 102 cm for men), dyslipidemia (triglycerides $\geq$ 150 mg/dL or HDL cholesterol $<$ 40 mg/dL in men, $<$50 mg/dL in women), and insulin resistance (fasting glucose $>$ 110 mg/dL). The increase in risk associated with this syndrome is fourfold for fatal coronary heart disease, twofold for cardiovascular fatality, and ninefold for developing diabetes [48]. Metabolic markers of insulin resistance (hyperglycemia, hyperinsulinemia, hypertriglyceridemia, high low-density lipids [LDL], and low high-density lipoprotein [HDL]) also predict mortality [49]. Obesity (body mass index [BMI] $>$ 25 kg/m^2) is associated with an increased risk for the development of posttransplant diabetes, hypertension, and hyperlipidemia [50]. Furthermore, obesity has been associated with greater graft loss because of an increased tendency for poorer response to antirejection therapy (acute steroid resistance), and a greater incidence of chronic allograft nephropathy. Diabetic patients with dyslipidemic profiles, eg, low HDL, high LDL, or high triglyceride levels, are a grave concern because of the additive risk for subsequent cardiovascular events [51].

Based on the review in the preceding paragraphs, it is clear that diabetes, hypertension, and hyperlipidemia are independent risk factors for adverse cardiovascular events after lung transplant, thus highlighting the importance of risk assessment, modification, and treatment of these comorbid conditions to avoid posttransplant cardiovascular morbidity and mortality.

Guidelines for managing diabetes, hypertension, and hyperlipidemia

While precise guidance for the diagnosis and management of diabetes, hypertension, and hyperlipidemia after transplant is lacking, expert panels suggest more aggressive target goals for blood pressure, glucose, and lipids in persons of high-risk groups (ie, those with compelling indications, including transplant recipients) [52]. The newest guidelines emphasize that previously borderline levels of glucose intolerance, pre-hypertension, and elevated lipids are now known to have significant risks associated with them and stress the benefits of instituting early risk assessment and modification strategies for individuals in the "pre" morbid stages because they are at great risk for progression to actual diabetes, hypertension, and hyperlipidemia (Table 2).

Guidelines for managing diabetes after transplantation include lower diagnostic thresholds for impaired glucose tolerance and diabetes to a fasting glucose of 110 to 126 mg/dL and 126 to 140 mg/dL, respectively [9]. The rationale for these changes was to identify individuals at high risk for developing diabetes and its adverse effects earlier. The term "pre-diabetes" is now used to refer to the group whose glucose levels do not meet the criteria for diabetes, but who cannot be considered normal because of impaired glucose tolerance [9]. Although at pre-diabetes levels, glucose levels are below diabetic thresholds, these recipients have a higher risk for the development of diabetes and cardiovascular complications, thus early diagnosis and treatment are essential. A1C levels (glycosylated hemoglobin, previously termed

Table 2
Criteria for staging of comorbid conditions

Diabetes glucose in mg/dL	Normal[a]	Pre-diabetes		Diabetes
	FPG < 110 OGT 2h < 140	Impaired glucose tolerance or fasting glucose FPG ≥ 110 < 126 or OGT 2h ≥140 < 200		FPG ≥ 126 any plasma glucose ≥ 200
Hypertension blood pressure in mm Hg	**Normal** SBP < 120 DBP < 80	**Pre-hypertension[a]** SBP 120–139 DBP 80–89	**Stage I hypertension** SBP 140–159 DBP 90–99	**Stage II hypertension** SBP > 160 DBP > 100
Hyperlipidemia lipid values in mg/dL	**Normal[a]** LDL < 100 TC < 200 TG < 150	**Borderline Pre-lipidemia** LDL 100–159 TC 200–239 TG 150–199	**High** LDL 160–189 TC 200–239 TG 200–499	**Very High** LDL >190 TC ≥ 240 TG ≥ 500

Compiled from guidelines for managing diabetes [9], hypertension [68] and hyperlipidemia [11].

Abbreviations: DBP, diastolic blood pressure; FPG, Fasting plasma glucose; LDL, low-density lipids; OGT, oral glucose tolerance test; SBP, systolic blood pressure; TC, total cholesterol; TG, triglyceride.

[a] Target goals for transplant and other high-risk groups: FPG ≤ 110; OGT ≤ 140 [56]; BP 130/80 [68]; LDL ≤ 70 [11].

Hb A_{1c}) are used to monitor recipients' response to therapy; target A1C levels of less than 6.5 are now recommended [53].

Based on the rate of cardiovascular adverse events noted in patients with borderline normal blood pressure (pre-hypertension) and the likelihood of increased blood pressure as one ages, the Seventh Report of the Joint National Committee on the Prevention, Detection, Evaluation, and Treatment of High Blood Pressure (JNC 7) now recommends early treatment of hypertension with blood pressures less than 130/80 mm Hg recommended for high-risk groups, including transplant recipients, such as those with other comorbidities or receiving immunosuppression [40].

According to Adult Treatment Panel III (ATP III) recommendations [11], all patients with lipid abnormalities for LDL, HDL, or triglycerides should be treated based on evidence of increasing risk for atherosclerotic adverse events at levels previously considered borderline normal. An LDL cholesterol level of less than 100 mg/dL is optimal; therefore, ATP III specifies an LDL cholesterol less than 100 mg/dL as the goal of therapy in secondary prevention. This goal is supported by trials with both clinical and angiographic endpoints and by prospective epidemiological studies. However, ATP III adds a call for more intensive LDL-lowering therapy to less than 70 mg/dL in certain high-risk groups [11], such as persons with diabetic renal dysfunction and those receiving drugs that increase LDL cholesterol and decrease HDL cholesterol (eg, immunosuppressants).

Recommendations for management of comorbidities before transplantation

Screening

A number of characteristics appear to predispose patients to the development of the immunosuppression-induced comorbid conditions after transplant. Not surprisingly, the strongest predictors include the presence of preexisting glucose intolerance, diabetes, obesity, hypertension or hyperlipidemia, or a positive family history for any of these conditions [54]. A complete medical and family history should be taken from all lung transplant candidates. Lung transplant candidates should be assessed for features of the metabolic syndrome, eg, blood pressure, obesity, LDL and HDL levels, and other cardiovascular risk factors (eg, smoking), as these factors raise the risk of developing posttransplant cardiovascular disease.

Screening also includes detecting previously undiagnosed diabetes, hypertension, or hyperlipidemia. A fasting plasma glucose (FPG) should be measured at regular intervals during the period that candidates are awaiting transplantation. For screening purposes, even candidates with normal FPG levels (<6.1 mmol/L or 110 mg/dL) should receive an oral glucose tolerance test [55] at both 0 and 2 hours post-challenge because it is more predictive of increased risk of cardiovascular morbidity and mortality than FPG testing, particularly in people with impaired glucose tolerance [56]. Patients identified with pre-diabetes (impaired glucose tolerance or fasting glucose) before transplantation should be observed closely for the development of new-onset diabetes after transplantation (see Table 2).

An accurate measurement of blood pressure is the mainstay of detecting hypertension [10]. The auscultatory method should be used to measure blood pressure after the patient has sat quietly for at least 5 minutes, in a chair (rather than an examining table), with feet on the floor and arm supported at heart level [57]. Two measurements should be taken and the average recorded with verification in the opposite arm. Data from epidemiological studies have also demonstrated that elevations in resting heart rate and reduced heart rate variability are associated with higher cardiovascular risk [58]. Therapy for patients with blood pressures above 130/80 mm Hg, the goal for persons in high-risk groups including lung transplant recipients, begins with lifestyle modifications (see Table 2), but if the blood pressure goal is not achieved, antihypertensive therapy should be initiated. Normotensive patients should be assessed at 6-month intervals. Patients in the pre-hypertension stage should be evaluated every 3 months to ensure that the target blood pressure is maintained; patients with stage I or II hypertension should return for follow-up evaluation and adjustment of treatment at least monthly until control is achieved.

A complete fasting lipoprotein profile (total cholesterol, LDL and HDL cholesterol, and triglycerides) is initially performed to determine risk for posttransplant hyperlipidemia. Risk factors considered in addition to the

LDL cholesterol level include the presence of preexisting cardiovascular disease or diabetes, and any of the following: age (men > 45 years; women > 55 years), stage I or II hypertension or receiving antihypertensive therapy, low HDL (< 40 mg/dL), history of cardiovascular disease in first-degree relative (males ≤ 55 years; females ≤ 65 years), and cigarette smoking (although lung transplant candidates cannot be current smokers). Any candidate with an elevated LDL or other form of hyperlipidemia should undergo further assessment to rule out conditions such as diabetes or thyroid, hepatic, or renal abnormalities that cause secondary dyslipidemia. Patients with elevated LDL cholesterol are initially treated by encouraging lifestyle changes, particularly emphasizing reduction in saturated fat and increasing fiber and exercise. Patients should be seen again in 6 weeks to evaluate LDL response; if elevations in LDL persist, plant stanols/sterols are added. If after another 6-week trial period, LDL goal (<100 mg/dL) is not achieved, transplant patients who are also candidates for drug treatment and lipid-lowing therapy should not be delayed. With moderately elevated triglycerides, the primary aim is still to achieve target LDL cholesterol levels, but borderline high triglycerides (150 to 199 mg/dL) warrant aggressive weight reduction and increased physical activity. With high triglyceride levels (200 to 499 mg/dL), cholesterol levels become secondary, and triglyceride levels drive therapy.

Nursing implications

First-line treatment for these comorbid conditions is lifestyle modification; however, because the likelihood of developing immunosuppressant-induced diabetes, hypertension, and hyperlipidemia is so high after lung transplant, all transplant candidates should be counseled about weight control, nutrition, and exercise as soon as possible. Healthy dietary and exercise habits decrease cardiovascular risk by postponing the onset of these conditions and enhancing drug efficacy. This is especially important for transplant candidates with any of the premorbid conditions. In overweight persons without other risk factors, weight loss of as little as 10 pounds (4.5 kg) reduced blood pressure and/or prevented hypertension, so transplant candidates should be counseled about maintaining ideal body weight or weight reduction [59].

A diet rich in fruits, vegetables, and low-fat dairy products with a reduced content of simple sugars, dietary cholesterol, and saturated and total fat is recommended. The use of plant stanols/sterols and viscous (soluble) fiber is encouraged as therapeutic dietary options to enhance reduction of LDL cholesterol. Referral to a nutritionist for counseling about specific dietary restrictions should be considered. Alcohol intake is discouraged, but for recipients who choose to consume alcoholic beverages, intake should be limited to < 1 ounce for men and 0.5 ounces for woman per day.

An exercise program designed for persons with cardiopulmonary disorders should be considered for all patients, even those with physical limitations. The intent is to optimize physical functioning while waiting for transplantation and to reduce the deconditioning that often accompanies major surgery and prolonged hospitalization. Although all lung candidates are required to stop smoking to be eligible for transplant, recipients with a previous smoking history should be strongly counseled to remain non-smokers for a variety of health reasons, including overall cardiovascular risk reduction.

Recommendations for management of comorbidities after transplantation

Selecting appropriate immunosuppressive therapy

While the effects of various immunosuppressive agents differ, they all contribute to the development of these comorbid conditions to some degree. The aim of individualizing the antirejection regimen is to balance effective immunosuppression with comorbidity risk reduction. Pretransplant risk factors should be used to tailor the initial selection of the antirejection agents to avoid worsening preexisting diabetes, hypertension, or hyperlipidemia or promoting the development of a condition to which the recipient is particularly susceptible. Typical immunosuppression regimen after lung transplant is composed of a calcineurin inhibitor, either tacrolimus or cyclosporine, plus a purine synthesis antagonist (mycophenolic acid derivative or proliferation signal inhibitor), and prednisone. The development of new-onset diabetes, hypertension, or hyperlipidemia may warrant changing agents because immunosuppressive drugs vary in their impact on glucose tolerance, blood pressure, and lipid metabolism effects.

Corticosteroids are associated with the highest risk for new-onset diabetes after transplantation [60,61]. Steroid-sparing immunosuppression regimens have been successful in controlling rejection in recipients of other solid organs, namely kidney [62], heart [63], and liver [64]; however, attempts to reduce the use of prednisone after lung transplantation have been unsuccessful in preventing rejection [25]. The calcineurin inhibitors also have diabetogenic effects. Evidence suggests that tacrolimus has greater diabetogenicity than cyclosporine, particularly in pediatric recipients and recipients of African decent [29,65]. Yet tacrolimus tends to be associated with better serum lipid profiles than those seen with cyclosporine-based regimens [37–39]. Changing tacrolimus-treated patients who develop new-onset diabetes to cyclosporine may improve glucose regulation, while conversion from cyclosporine to tacrolimus is generally associated with improved serum lipid profiles. When glucose or lipid control cannot be established even after a change in therapy, the primary immunosuppressant may be discontinued altogether. Thus, antirejection therapy relies on secondary immunosuppressants and prednisone. Change in immunosuppression strategies to reduce serious cardiovascular comorbid states necessitates close monitoring for rejection of lung transplant.

Treating to target

The goal of treating diabetes, hypertension, and hyperlipidemia is to reduce cardiovascular morbidity and mortality. Management of lung recipients should aim toward tight glycemic, blood pressure, and lipid control as there is evidence from the general population that treating to target can substantially lower the potential for cardiovascular complications [56,66,67]. Target values for posttransplant glucose, blood pressure, and lipids (highlighted with an asterisk in Table 2) are lower than those for the general population because posttransplant immunosuppression and its concomitant comorbidities, qualify as compelling indications, thus placing them in the high-risk category [56,68]. Interventions to achieve optimal control vary with each recipient, but the presence of co-occurring conditions (such as diabetes and hypertension, or diabetes and hyperlipidemia) requires more intensive therapy. When desired control is not achieved with initial therapy, more aggressive or combination therapy approaches are used.

Elevations of LDL cholesterol are the primary target of cholesterol-lowering therapy, although moderate elevations of triglycerides also warrant pharmacologic intervention after transplant because of their increased risk for lipid dysfunction. Transplant recipients are prescribed more intensive LDL-lowering treatments to achieve the lower target of LDL less than 70 mg/dL and triglycerides of less than 150 mg/dL. Statin therapy is beneficial even for persons with low LDL cholesterol levels who have a history of cardiovascular disease [66,69]. Additionally, the use of statins early after kidney [70] and heart transplantation [71] has been shown to improve survival, presumably by reducing cardiovascular complications. More recently, the immunosuppressive benefits of statin use have been recognized, and the initiation of statins early after lung transplantation to control lipidemia has been shown to improve function and survival of lung allografts [41,42]. Statins and calcineurin inhibitors are metabolized similarly, thus potential drug interactions need to be carefully considered when dosing. All fibrates (with the exception of gemfibrozil), the primary therapy for people with markedly elevated triglyceride levels (>6.8 mmol/L or 500 mg/dL), have been shown to reduce blood cyclosporine levels [72]; therefore, these agents may require adjustments in cyclosporine dose and should be used with caution in recipients with renal insufficiency. Use of statins with fibrates is contraindicated; therefore, combination therapies warrant particular consideration.

None of the current antihypertensive agents are contraindicated in transplant patients. However, angiotensin-converting enzyme inhibitors (ACEIs) are typically prescribed initially to try to achieve a target blood pressure of less than 130/80 mm Hg. Care should be taken when giving ACEIs and other antihypertensive agents during the first 6 months after transplant in the setting of excessive cyclosporine or tacrolimus levels and aspirin use should be considered to further reduce the risk of cardiovascular events.

Ongoing monitoring

All recipients, regardless of diabetes status, should routinely undergo fasting plasma glucose (FPG) testing weekly for the first month, every 3 months for the first year, and annually thereafter to detect the onset of abnormal glucose regulation [56]. If the FPG level is more than 6.1 mmol/L or 110 mg/dL an oral glucose tolerance test (OGTT) is required to further assess for the development of diabetes. A1C monitoring should be performed simultaneously with the FPG schedule beginning at the 3-month posttransplant evaluation. This delay is necessary because perioperative blood transfusions render the test invalid until new hemoglobin is constituted.

Ongoing monitoring of blood pressure is crucial after transplantation. Even normotensive recipients should have their blood pressure assessed at monthly intervals. Patients in the prehypertension stage should also be evaluated monthly to ensure that the target blood pressure is maintained; patients with stage I or II hypertension should return for follow-up evaluation and adjustment of treatment at least monthly.

Lipid profiles should be monitored frequently in lung recipients (at least every 6 weeks after transplant) as long as values remain at optimal levels. Variation from target levels requires an increased frequency of monitoring and adjustment of therapies to achieve target goals.

Self-monitoring

Patient self-monitoring of blood glucose is an essential component of the therapeutic plan of recipients who are taking oral hypoglycemic agents or insulin, and may also be useful for recipients whose diabetes is controlled with diet alone [73]. The frequency of home testing will vary between individuals but should be sufficient to provided feedback to optimize therapy.

Self-monitoring of blood pressure at home is used to assess differences between clinic and out-of-clinic measurements and to detect gradual trends and response to therapies between clinic visits. Home devices should be examined for accuracy so clinic and home comparisons will be valid. Patients should be provided with a target goal for blood pressure, as well as given instructions regarding the level of blood pressure abnormality to report to the transplant center between follow-up visits.

Nursing implications

Nurses play a crucial role in educating lung recipients about the benefits of lifestyle changes and adhering to prescribed treatment regimens. Numerous studies have documented the difficulty patients, including transplant recipients [74–77], experience adhering to healthy lifestyles [78–81] and regimens to control diabetes [82,83], hypertension [84–86], and hyperlipidemia [87–90]. Furthermore, the development of concomitant comorbidities after lung transplant places additional burdens on patients as they attempt to adhere to a complex medical regimen.

Evidence-based guidelines for treating each of the three comorbid conditions have been developed and their use proven to be effective in reducing subsequent cardiovascular morbidity and mortality in the general population. The current approach to treating these conditions after lung transplantation is to parcel the management to specialists in the specific condition. However, reliance on separate protocols to manage conditions that typically co-occur may be less than optimal, particularly when one considers the additive effects of having multiple comorbidities (diabetes, hypertension, and lipidemia) on the cardiovascular risk profile, the complexity of the medical regimen, and the potential for adverse interactions between therapies.

It is our contention that to optimize the risk profile for cardiovascular morbidity and mortality after lung transplantation, a more integrated approach to the assessment and treatment of these conditions is needed and nurses are well suited to lead such efforts. Therefore, we are currently in the process of designing a nursing intervention that combines the individual treatment guidelines for diabetes, hypertension, and hyperlipidemia with theoretical knowledge about behavior change, and strategies to individualize care and enhance patient adherence, into one integrated risk assessment and management protocol for use with lung transplant patients.

Summary

The degree of impairment, posttransplant date of onset, and rate of progression for diabetes, hypertension, and hyperlipidemia differ substantially among individual lung recipients, emphasizing the importance of early and ongoing risk assessment, modification, and treatment. Because of their higher risk for developing comorbidities than other transplant recipients, the ability to predict a lung recipient's risk for developing multiple comorbidities after transplantation would be of benefit in identifying those who may need more intensive monitoring, risk-factor intervention, or individualized treatment. Studies suggest that early screening, appropriate assessment, and risk modification of patients before and after transplantation can minimize the risks for developing these comorbid conditions. Moreover, nursing interventions that promote ongoing assessments, early detection, and appropriate management of lung recipients who have developed these comorbidities may reduce the potential for subsequent cardiovascular adverse events. Although some of these factors may not be modifiable, the risks may be additive. Therefore, the assessment of risk should play a significant role in the ongoing surveillance and management of lung transplant recipients.

Adopting an integrated approach to managing these comorbid conditions simultaneously both before and after lung transplantation will likely improve adherence to the complex regimen and reduce lung recipients' risks for future cardiovascular morbidity and mortality.

References[A,B]

[1] Organ Procurement and Transplantation Network. Annual report of the U.S. organ procurement and transplantation network and the scientific registry of transplant recipients. Transplant Data 1994–2007. 2007. Available at: www.optn.org/latestData/rptData.asp. Accessed June 28, 2007, B.

[2] DeMeo DL, Ginns LC. Lung transplantation at the turn of the century. Annu Rev Med 2001;52:185–201, B.

[3] Girgis RE, Tu I, Berry GJ, et al. Risk factors for the development of obliterative bronchiolitis after lung transplantation. J Heart Lung Transplant 1996;15(12):1200–8, B.

[4] Trulock EP, Edwards LB, Taylor DO, et al. Registry of the international society for heart and lung transplantation: twenty-second official adult lung & heart-lung transplant report—2005. J Heart Lung Transplant 2005;24(8):956–67, B.

[5] Studer SM, Levy RD, McNeil K, et al. Lung transplant outcomes: a review of survival, graft function, physiology, health-related quality of life and cost-effectiveness. Eur Respir J 2004; 24(4):674–85, B.

[6] Organ Procurement and Transplantation Network. 2003 Annual report of the U.S. registry of transplant recipients and transplant data 1988–2003. 2003; Available at: www.optn.org/latestData/rptData.asp. Accessed November 24, 2003.

[7] Bernardo JF, McCauley J. Drug therapy in transplant recipients: special considerations in the elderly with co-morbid conditions. Drugs Aging 2004;21(5):323–48, B.

[8] American Diabetes Association. Diagnosis and classification of diabetes mellitus. Diabetes Care 2005;28(Suppl):S37–42, B.

[9] Davidson JA, Wilkinson A, Dantal J, et al. New-onset diabetes after transplantation. 2003 International consensus guidelines. Transplantation 2003;75(10):SS3–24, A.

[10] Pickering TG, Hall JE, Appel LJ, et al. Recommendations for blood pressure measurements in humans and experimental animals. Part I: blood pressure measurement in humans. Hypertension 2005;45(2):142–61, A.

[11] National Cholesterol Education Committee. Third report of the national cholesterol education program (NCEP) expert panel on detection, evaluation, and treatment of high blood cholesterol in adults (Adult Treatment Panel III): final report. Circulation 2002;106(25):3143–421, A.

[12] Trulock EP, Edwards LB, Taylor DO, et al. Registry of the international society for heart and lung transplantation: twenty-third official adult lung and heart-lung transplantation report. J Heart Lung Transplant 2006;25(8):880–92, B.

[13] Aker S, Ivens K, Grabensee B, et al. Cardiovascular risk factors and diseases after renal transplantation. Int Urol Nephrol 1998;30(6):777–88, B.

[14] Rabkin JM, Corless CL, Rosen HR, et al. Immunosuppression impact on long-term cardiovascular complications after liver transplantation. Am J Surg 2002;183(5):595–9, B.

[15] Guckelberger O, Mutzke F, Gianemann M, et al. Validation of cardiovascular risk scores in a liver transplant population. Liver Transpl 2006;12(3):394–401, B.

[16] Sekine Y, Waddell TK, Matte-Martyn A. Risk quantification of early outcome after lung transplantation: donor, recipient, operative, and post-transplant parameters. J Heart Lung Transplant 2004;23(1):96–104, B.

[A] Grade A = RCT and meta-analyses.
[B] Grade B = other evidence.

[17] Kaza CS, Deitz JF, Kern JA, et al. Coronary risk stratification in patients with end-stage lung disease. J Heart Lung Transplant 2002;21(3):334–9, B.

[18] Markell M. New-onset diabetes mellitus in transplant patients: pathogenesis, complications, and management. Am J Kidney Dis 2004;43(6):953–65, B.

[19] Montori VM, Dinneen SF, Gorman CA, et al. The impact of planned care and a diabetes electronic management system on community-based diabetes care. Diabetes Care 2002; 25(11):1952–7, A.

[20] Dmitrewski J, Krentz AJ, Mayer AD, et al. Metabolic and hormonal effects of tacrolimus (FK506) or cyclosporin immunosuppression following renal transplantation. Diabetes Obes Metab 2001;3(4):287–92, B.

[21] Fellstrom B. Risk factors for and management of post-transplantation cardiovascular disease. BioDrugs 2001;15(4):261–78, B.

[22] Shitrit D, Rahamimov R, Gidon S, et al. Use of sirolimus and low-dose calcineurin inhibitor in lung transplant recipients with renal impairment: results of a controlled pilot study. Kidney Int 2005;67(4):1471–5, A.

[23] World Health Organization. Definition, diagnosis and classification of diabetes mellitus and its complications. 2004; Available at: www.nzgg.org.nz/library/gl_complete/diabetes/who_report_diabets_diagnosis-.pdf. Accessed August 16, 2005, B.

[24] Hjelmesaeth J, Hartmann A, Kofstad J, et al. Tapering off prednisolone and cyclosporine the first year after renal transplantation: the effect on glucose tolerance. Nephrol Dial Transplant 2001;16(4):829–35, B.

[25] Walczak DA, Calvert D, Jarzembowski TM, et al. Increased risk of post-transplant diabetes mellitus despite early steroid discontinuation in hispanic kidney transplant recipients. Clin Transplant 2005;19(4):527–31, B.

[26] Jindal RM, Hjelmesaeth J. Impact and management of post transplant diabetes mellitus. Transplantation 2000;70(11):S58–63, B.

[27] Cosio FG, Pesavento TE, Sei K, et al. Post-transplant diabetes mellitus: increasing incidence in renal allograft recipients transplanted in recent years. Kidney Int 2001;59(2):732–7, B.

[28] Sumrani NB, Delaney V, Ding Z, et al. Diabetes after renal transplantation in the cyclosporine era: an analysis of risk factors. Transplantation 1991;51(2):343–7, B.

[29] Kasiske BL, Snyder JJ, Gilbertson D, et al. Diabetes mellitus after transplantation in the United States. Am J Transplant 2003;3(2):178–85, B.

[30] Lindholm A, Albrechtsen D, Frodin L, et al. Ischemic heart disease: major cause of death and graft loss after renal transplantation in Scandinavia. Transplantation 1995;60(5): 451–7, B.

[31] Grundy SM, Benjamin IJ, Burke GL, et al. Prevention conference VI: diabetes and cardiovascular disease: executive summary: conference proceeding for healthcare professionals form a special writing group of the American Heart Association. Circulation 2000; 101(13):1629–31, B.

[32] Rutherford RM, Fisher AJ, Hilton C, et al. Functional status and quality of life in patients surviving 10 years after lung transplantation. Am J Transplant 2005;5:1099–104, B.

[33] Morrison RJ, Short HD, Noon GP, et al. Hypertension and lung transplantation. J Heart Lung Transplant 1993;12(6):928–31, B.

[34] Canzello VJ. Management of post-transplant hypertension. In: Izzo JL, Black HR, editors. Hypertension primer: the essentials of high blood pressure: basic science, population science, and clinical management. Philadelphia: Lippincott Williams & Wilkins; 2003. p. 519–22, B.

[35] Miller JA, Curtis JR, Sochett EB. Relationship between diurnal blood pressure, renal hemodynamic function, and the renin-angiotensin system in type 1 diabetes. Diabetes 2003;52(6): 1806–11, A.

[36] Cohen F. Measurement in coping, in stress and health. In: Kasl SV, Cooper CL, editors. Issues in research methodology. Winchester (VA): Wiley; 1987. p. 283–305, B.

[37] Artz MA, Boots JMM, Ligtenberg G, et al. Randomized conversion from cyclosporine to tacrolimus in renal transplant patients: improved lipid profile and unchanged plasma homocysteine levels. Transplant Proc 2002;34(5):1793–4, A.

[38] Manu M, Tanabe K, Tokumoto I, et al. Impact of tacrolimus on hyperlipidiemia after renal transplantation. Transplant Proc 2000;32(7):1736–8, B.

[39] Plosker GL, Foster RH. Tacrolimus: a further update of its pharmacology and therapeutic use in the management of organ transplantation. Drugs Aging 2000;59(2):323–89, B.

[40] Heeneman S, Donners MM, Bai L, et al. Drug-induced immunomodulation to affect the development and progression of atherosclerosis: a new opportunity? Expert Rev Cardiovasc Ther 2007;5(2):345–64, B.

[41] Johnson BA, Iacono AT, Zeevi A, et al. Statin use is associated with improved function and survival of lung allografts. Am J Respir Crit Care Med 2003;167(9):1271–8, B.

[42] Kobashigawa JA, Moriguchi JD, Laks H, et al. Ten-year follow-up of a randomized trial of pravastatin in heart transplant patients. J Heart Lung Transplant 2005;24(11):1736–40, A.

[43] Silverborn M, Jeppsson A, Martensson G, et al. New-onset cardiovascular risk factors in lung transplant recipients. J Heart Lung Transplant 2005;24(10):1536–43, B.

[44] Benhamou PY, Penfornis A. Natural history, prognosis and management of transplantation-induced diabetes-mellitus. Diabetes Metab 2002;28(3):166–75, B.

[45] Davis TM, Millins H, Stratton IM, et al. Risk factors for stroke in type 2 diabetes mellitus: United Kingdom prospective diabetes study (UKPDS). Arch Intern Med 1999;159(10): 1097–103, B.

[46] Fagan TC, Sowers J. Type 2 diabetes mellitus: greater cardiovascular risks and greater benefits of therapy. Arch Intern Med 1999;159(10):1033–4, B.

[47] Ford ES, Giles WH, Dietz WH. Prevalence of the metabolic syndrome among US adults: findings from the third national health and nutrition examination survey. JAMA 2002; 287(3):356–9, B.

[48] Wilson PWF, D'Agastino RB, Parise H, et al. The metabolic syndrome as a precursor of cardiovascular disease and type 2 diabetes mellitus. Diabetes 2002;51:A242, B.

[49] Valantine H, Rickenbacker P. Metabolic abnormalities characteristic of dysmetabolic syndrome predict the development of transplant coronary artery disease: a prospective study. Circulation 2001;103(17):2144–52, B.

[50] van den Ham EC, Kooman JP. Relation between steroid dose, body composition, and physical activity in renal transplant patients. Transplantation 2000;69(8):1591–8, B.

[51] Drown DJ. Dyslipidemic profile of the diabetic: a grave concern. Prog Cardiovasc Nurs 2005;20(3):126, B.

[52] Chobanian AV, Bakris GL, Black HR, et al. JNC 7: Seventh report of the joint national committee on prevention, detection, evaluation, and treatment of blood pressure. Hypertension 2003;42(6):1206–52, A.

[53] Diabetic Complications, DCCT. The effect of intensive treatment of diabetes on the development and progression of long-term complications in insulin-dependent diabetes mellitus. N Engl J Med 1993;329(14):977–86, A.

[54] Alberti KG, Zimmet PZ. Definition, diagnosis and classification of diabetes mellitus and its complications: provisional report of a WHO consultation. Diabet Med 1998;15(7): 539–53, B.

[55] Boehler A, Vogt P, Zollinger A, et al. Prospective study of the value of transbronchial lung biopsy after lung transplantation. Eur Respir J 1996;9(4):658–62, B.

[56] Wilkinson A, Davidson J, Dotta F, et al. Guidelines for the treatment and management of new-onset diabetes after transplantation. Clin Transplant 2005;19:291–8, A.

[57] World Health League. Measuring blood pressure 2003. Available at: http://www.mco.edu/org/whl/bloodpre.html. Accessed January 21, 2007, B.

[58] Kannel WB, Kannel C, Paffenbarger RS, et al. Heart rate and cardiovascular mortality: the Framingham study. Am Heart J 1987;113(6):1489–94, B.

[59] National Institutes of Health. Clinical guidelines on the identification, evaluation, and treatment of overweight and obesity in adults: the evidence report. Obes Res 1998;6(S2): 51S–209S, A.

[60] Baid S, Cosimi AB, Farrell ML, et al. Posttransplant diabetes mellitus in liver transplant recipients: risk factors, temporal relationship with hepatitis C virus allograft hepatitis, and impact on mortality. Transplantation 2001;72(6):1066–72, B.

[61] Depczynski B, Daly B, Campbell LV, et al. Predicting the occurrence of diabetes mellitus in recipients of heart transplants. Diabet Med 2000;17(1):15–9, B.

[62] Hricik DE, Knauss TC, Bodziak KA, et al. Withdrawal of steroid therapy in African American kidney transplant recipients. Transplantation 2003;76(6):938–42, B.

[63] Felkel TO, Smith AL, Reichenspurner HC. Survival and incidence of acute rejection in heart transplant recipients undergoing successful withdrawal of steroid therapy. J Heart Lung Transplant 2002;21(5):530–9, B.

[64] Pirenne J, Aerts R, Koshiba T. Steroid-free immunosuppression during and after liver transplantation—a 3 year follow-up report. Clin Transplant 2003;17(3):177–82, B.

[65] Al-Uzri A, Stablein DM, Cohn R. Post-transplant diabetes mellitus in pediatric renal transplant recipients: a report of the North American pediatric renal transplant cooperative study (NAPRTCS). Transplantation 2001;72(6):1020–4, B.

[66] Nissen SE, Tuzcu EM, Schoenhagen P, et al. Effect of intensive compared with moderate lipid-lowering therapy on progression of coronary atherosclerosis: a randomized controlled trial. JAMA 2004;291(9):1071–80, A.

[67] Altunkan S, Yildiz S, Azer S. Blood pressure-measuring devices: a comparative study of accuracy with standard auscultatory method for using a mercury monometer. Blood Press Monit 2002;7(5):281–4, B.

[68] National High Blood Pressure Education Program Coordinating Committee, JNC 7. The seventh report of the joint national committee on prevention, detection, evaluation and treatment of high blood pressure. JAMA 2003;289(19):2560–72, A.

[69] Cannon CP, Steinberg BA, Murphy SA, et al. Meta-analysis of cardiovascular outcomes trials comparing intensive versus moderate statin therapy. J Am Coll Cardiol 2006;48(3): 438–45, A.

[70] Cosio FG, Pesavento TE, Pelletier RP. Patient survival after renal transplantation III: the effects of statins. Am J Kidney Dis 2002;40(3):638–43, A.

[71] Wenke K, Meiser B, Thierry J, et al. Simvastatin initiated early after heart transplantation: 8-year prospective experience. Circulation 2003;107(1):93–7, A.

[72] Boissonnat P, Salen P, Guidollet J, et al. The long-term effects of the lipid-lowering agent fenofibrate in hyperlipidemic heart transplant recipients. Transplantation 1994;58(2):245–7, B.

[73] Expert Committee on the Diagnosis and Classification of Diabetes Mellitus. Report of the expert committee on the diagnosis and classification of diabetes mellitus. Diabetes Care 2003;26(Suppl 1):S5–20, B.

[74] Dew MA, Dunbar-Jacob J, Switzer GE, et al. Adherence to the medical regimen in transplantation. In: Rodrigue JR, editor. Biopsychosocial perspectives on transplantation. New York: Kluwer Academic/Plenum Publishers; 2001. p. 93–124. B.

[75] Dew MA, DiMartini AF, De Vito Dabbs A, et al. Rates and risk factors for nonadherence to the medical regimen after adult solid organ transplantation. Transplantation 2007;83(7): 858–73, A.

[76] Dobbels F, Vanhaecke J, Desmyttere A, et al. Prevalence and correlates of self-reported pretransplant nonadherence with medication in heart, liver, and lung transplant candidates. Transplantation 2005;79(11):1588–95, B.

[77] Josephson MA. Improving medication adherence in transplant recipients: managing physical side effects of immunosuppression. Medscape Transplant Web MD 2005;6(2). Available at: http://www.medscape.com/viewarticle/508880. Accessed December 12, 2006, B.

[78] DiMatteo MR. Variations in patients' adherence to medical recommendations: a quantitative review of 50 years of research. Med Care 2004;42(3):200–9, A.

[79] Leong J, Molassiotis A, Marsh H. Adherence to health recommendations after a cardiac rehabilitation program in post-myocardial infarction patients: the role of health beliefs, locus of control and psychological status. Clinical Effectiveness in Nursing 2004;8(1): 26–38, B.

[80] Vitolins MZ, Rand CS, Rapp SR, et al. Measuring adherence to behavioral and medical interventions. Control Clin Trials 2000;21(5S):188S–94S, B.

[81] World Health Organization. Adherence to long-term therapies: evidence for action. 2003. Available at: http://www.who.int/topics/patient_adherence/en/. Accessed April 11, 2007, B.

[82] Sigurdardottir AK. Self-care in diabetes: model of factors affecting self-care. J Clin Nurs 2005;14:301–14, A.

[83] Vermeire E, Wens J, Van Royen P, et al. Interventions for improving adherence to treatment recommendations in people with type 2 diabetes mellitus [Online]. Cochrane Database Syst Rev 2005;2:CD003638, A.

[84] DiMatteo MR, Giordani PJ, Lepper HS, et al. Patient adherence and medical treatment outcomes: a meta-analysis. Med Care 2002;40(9):794–811, A.

[85] Domino FJ. Improving adherence to treatment for hypertension. Am Fam Physician 2005; 71(11):2089–90, B.

[86] Weir MR, Maibach EW, Bakris GL, et al. Implications of a healthy lifestyle and medication analysis for improving hypertension control. Arch Intern Med 2000;160(4):481–90, B.

[87] Baird KK, Pierce LL. Adherence to cardiac therapy for men with coronary artery disease. Rehabil Nurs 2001;26(6):233–7, 243, 251, B.

[88] Becker DM, Allen JK. Improving compliance in your dyslipidemic patient: an evidence-based approach. J Am Acad Nurse Pract 2001;13(5):200–7, B.

[89] Senior V, Marteau TM, Weinman J, et al. Self-reported adherence to cholesterol-lowering medication in patients with familial hypercholesterolaemia: the role of illness perceptions. Cardiovasc Drugs Ther 2004;18(6):475–81, B.

[90] Stilley CS, Sereika S, Muldoon MF, et al. Psychological and cognitive function: Predictors of adherence with cholesterol lowering treatment. Ann Behav Med 2004;27(2):117–24, B.

NURSING
CLINICS
OF NORTH AMERICA

ELSEVIER
SAUNDERS

Nurs Clin N Am 43 (2008) 55–76

Respiratory and Cardiac Manifestations of Obstructive Sleep Apnea

Dorothy S. Lee, MSN, APRN BC[a,b,*]

[a]College of Nursing, Wayne State University, Detroit, MI 48202, USA
[b]Respiratory Physiology Laboratory B-4212, John D. Dingell Veterans Affairs Medical
Center 11-R, 4646 John R. Street, Detroit, MI 48201, USA

Obstructive sleep apnea hypopnea syndrome (OSAHS) is largely under-diagnosed in the general population, because as few as 20% of cases are symptomatic [1–4] and as many as 80% of all cases of OSAHS are unrecognized by primary care practitioners [1,5–7]. OSAHS is estimated to affect 4% of men and 2% of women in Western countries, with a male to female ratio of 2 to 1 [8–12]. Lack of symptoms reported by the patient should not minimize the importance of insidious underlying manifestations that occur within the respiratory and cardiovascular systems over time in untreated OSAHS [13]. These can lead to pathologic conditions, such as systemic hypertension, congestive heart failure, stroke, myocardial ischemia and infarction, pulmonary hypertension, and sudden death [3,4,11,12,14–16]. Moderate to severe OSAHS was associated with a 37% mortality rate during an 8-year study period [17]. Thus, it is critically important to identify and treat OSAHS patients early to avoid debilitating respiratory and cardiovascular manifestations.

OSAHS is defined as recurrent episodes of irregular breathing, characterized by the absence (apnea) or reduction (hypopnea) of airflow for more than 10 seconds in the presence of ventilatory efforts during sleep, along with an associated symptom (eg, excessive daytime sleepiness) [9,11,18–21]. The number of apneas and hypopneas per hours of sleep (ie, the apnea-hypopnea index [AHI]) is used to characterize the severity of the disorder. Apneas and hypopneas are accompanied by a decrease in arterial oxygen saturation (SaO_2) and an increase in arterial carbon dioxide levels ($PaCO_2$), terminating with arousal from sleep and re-establishment of airway patency [22]. Routine exposure to intermittent decreases in oxygen

* John D. Dingell Veteran's Affairs Medical Center 11-R, Respiratory Physiology Laboratory B-4212, 4646 John R. Street, Detroit, MI 48201.
  E-mail address: dorothy.lee1@va.gov

0029-6465/08/$ - see front matter © 2008 Elsevier Inc. All rights reserved.
doi:10.1016/j.cnur.2007.11.002
nursing.theclinics.com

and increases in carbon dioxide levels have been associated with oxidative stress, increased sympathetic activation, inflammation, endothelial dysfunction, and metabolic disturbance [23–27]. Repetitive sleep arousal leads to sleep fragmentation, manifested as excessive daytime sleepiness and other forms of neurocognitive dysfunction. These manifestations have been linked with motor vehicle and work-related accidents, diminished work performance, decreased school performance, and dissatisfaction with personal and social relationships [8,12,19,28,29]. Thus, OSAHS is a significant health care problem [30,31].

Historical view

OSAHS was first pathologically related to intermittent airway obstruction in 1965, simultaneously by Gastaut and colleagues [32] in France and Jung and Kuhlo [33] in Germany. Both groups likened the disorder to the rotund red-faced character Joe, described by Charles Dickens in *The Posthumous Papers of the Pickwick Club* (originally published in 1835). Joe was a boy who was obese and markedly somnolent, with a ruddy complexion, and this subsequently led to usage of the term "Pickwickian Syndrome." Today however, Pickwickian Syndrome specifically describes an individual with morbid obesity resulting in alveolar hypoventilation. This manifests as somnolence, secondary polycythemia, wakeful hypoventilation with hypercapnia and hypoxia, and pulmonary hypertension, which ultimately leads to right-sided heart failure.

Until 1981, the only recognized treatment for OSAHS was tracheostomy. However, the development of nasal continuous positive airway pressure (CPAP) proved to be an effective noninvasive therapy for the maintenance of airway patency [29,34]. Over the past three decades, the epidemiologic and clinical research conducted on OSAHS, with respect to associated morbidity and mortality, has ranked OSAHS as an increasingly significant health problem worthy of diagnosis and treatment [3,8,29,35,36].

Sleep-related breathing disorders

The *International Classification of Sleep Disorders*, version 2 was published to aid clinicians by consolidating detailed information regarding the classification of sleep disorders for diagnostic, epidemiologic, and research purposes [37,38]. OSAHS is classified under the spectrum of sleep-related breathing disorders (SBD), but is more specifically categorized under the heading of obstructive sleep apnea disorders because of the presence of upper airway collapse or narrowing, resulting in inadequate ventilation despite increased breathing effort [38]. OSAHS is considered a syndrome because it contains the obstructive sleep apnea and hypopnea component along with one or more accompanying daytime symptoms

[9,35]. The most commonly reported symptoms are excessive daytime somnolence, nonrestorative sleep, and fatigue [19]. An apnea-hypopnea index or AHI (number of occurrences per hour) of five or greater, with accompanying daytime somnolence, is indicative of OSAHS [14], although there are some adults with an AHI of five events per hour that do not experience symptoms.

Respiratory events that are not intense enough to meet the definition of apnea or hypopnea, but still result in arousal from sleep, are termed upper airway resistance events or respiratory effort related arousals. Upper airways resistance syndrome (UARS) does not have a separate diagnostic classification, as it is recognized as a milder manifestation of obstructive sleep apnea syndrome. Like OSAHS, UARS is manifested by events with increased inspiratory efforts and concomitant arousals, and a lack of recurrent apneas [19]. In UARS, the AHI is less than five per hour and oxygen desaturation does not occur during events [39]. However, subjective reports and objective evidence of excessive daytime sleepiness is prevalent.

Central sleep apnea syndromes differ from OSAHS: while there is cessation of breathing with central sleep apnea, there is no evidence of thoracic or abdominal efforts to breathe [13,19,40]. Central sleep apnea syndromes are the result of decreased neural output to the respiratory motor neurons [41], while obstructive sleep apnea is characterized by upper airway collapse during inspiration, along with neuromuscular efforts insufficient to restore airway patency. An AHI of 5 to fewer than 15 events per hour is characterized as mild OSAHS, 15 to 30 events per hour as moderate, and more than 30 events per hour as severe [12,19]. Habitual snoring, excessive daytime somnolence, and sleep fragmentation from frequent awakenings and arousals are common features of both central and obstructive apnea syndromes [3,6].

Epidemiology

In the 1990s, several robust epidemiologic studies were conducted to determine the prevalence of OSAHS. The Wisconsin Sleep Cohort Study examined a cohort of 602 middle-aged men and women, ranging from 30 to 60 years of age [11], and determined that 4% of men and 2% of women suffered from OSAHS. Sleep disordered breathing (SDB) without associated daytime somnolence has been found in 9% of women and 24% of men [11,42]. The Sleep Heart Health Study examined a cohort of 2,685 participants, ranging in age from 37 to 92 years old, to study sleep patterns and the prevalence of SDB [43]. SDB was present in 2% to 4% of middle-aged adults and 25% of elders.

More recent studies focusing on the prevalence of OSAHS have demonstrated that 20% of Caucasian nonobese adults with a body mass index of 25 kg/m^2 to 28 kg/m^2 suffer from mild OSAHS (AHI greater than or equal to 5), and 6% suffer from moderate OSAHS (AHI greater than or equal to 15) [11,12,35,44]. This cohort represents an unrecognized and undiagnosed population that does not match the typical profile, but are afflicted with OSAHS. Without identification, they will be subject to neurocognitive and cardiovascular health sequelae associated with untreated OSAHS.

Known risk factors

There are several known risk factors for the development of OSAHS, which include obesity, snoring, male gender, and alterations in craniofacial and oropharyngeal structures. The prevalence of OSAHS is known to increase with neck circumference and abdominal girth (waist-to-hip ratio) [29,36,45]. Increased fat deposition in the pharyngeal walls and reduction of tidal volume secondary to increased abdominal girth are believed to be partly responsible for the association between obesity and OSAHS [46–48].

Snoring is a well-established risk factor for OSAHS and has been associated with daytime sleepiness independent of the AHI [35,49]. Snoring is an involuntary vibratory sound resulting from a substantial decrease in the caliber of the oropharynx, creating turbulent airflow [50,51]. Oropharyngeal structures that may be involved in snoring include soft tissues of the palate, uvula, tonsils, base of the tongue, pharyngeal muscles, and the pharyngeal membranes [52]. Snoring is more common in men than women and has high association with obesity and daytime sleepiness [49,51].

Compared with the large-scale epidemiologic studies that estimate OSAHS affects 4% of men and 2% of women, clinic-based populations show a remarkably lower prevalence of women with OSAHS (approximately 5–8:1) [53]. Little is known as to the reason for the disparity in the clinic-based presentation. Perhaps in the clinic setting, OSAHS is considered a disease of men, with little recognition of its importance and prevalence among women to prompt screening.

In nonobese adults, OSAHS is linked with alterations in craniofacial and oropharyngeal structures [54–56]. Pharyngeal soft tissues [57], along with the position of the mandible and hyoid bone, may likewise diminish airway size and contribute to airway narrowing and occlusion [55].

Sleep

Normal sleep is a progression through a series of five sleep stages in cycles. Sleep is staged in epochs, or 30-second increments, and classified into two categories: nonrapid eye movement sleep (non-REM) and rapid eye movement (REM) sleep. Sleep is evaluated by electroencephalogram (EEG), which measures cortical electrical activity, electrooculogram (EOG), which measures eye movement during sleep, and a chin electromyogram (EMG), which measures skeletal muscle tone in the mental and submental areas of the chin [51,58]. EEG, EOG, and EMG are used to determine sleep stage, wakefulness, and arousal from sleep [59].

Non-REM sleep is further divided into four stages that increase in depth and unresponsiveness [60]. In Stage 1 sleep, the arousal threshold is low, such that sleep can be interrupted by the sound of a closing door, by calling the person's name, or by gently touching the person. Stage 1 sleep normally lasts about 2 to 7 minutes during the first cycle of sleep. It is considered a transition state that moves the person from wakefulness to sleep in cycles throughout the night. EEG signals denote a reduction in amplitude and frequency when compared with wakefulness signals. The EOG shows slow rolling eye movements, and the EMG reflects tonic activity that is slightly decreased from that of wakefulness [30]. An increase in percentage of Stage 1 sleep is associated with sleep disruption [61].

In Stage 2 sleep, the EEG waveforms are basically low volume voltage, with mixed frequency activity. Eye movements are often absent during this stage; however, there may be slow rolling eye movements at the onset of Stage 2. Low level tonic activity is observable in the EMG channel. Stage 2 lasts approximately 10 to 25 minutes in the first sleep cycle [60,61]. A stronger stimulus is required to awaken a person from Stage 2 sleep [30].

Stages 3 and 4 are often referred to as slow wave sleep, deep sleep, or delta sleep. The EEG signals show large prominent delta waves, with high amplitude and slow frequency [30]. Eye movements are absent; however, the EOG will register delta wave signals. Stage 3 is distinguished from Stage 4 by the amount of delta waves in the epoch [31]. EMG activity in both stages is tonic with low level activity. Stages 3 and 4 are jointly referred to as restorative sleep: that is, sleep associated with the feeling of awakening refreshed and well rested.

REM sleep is the stage of sleep associated with dreaming. The EEG waveform in this stage is low voltage with mixed frequency, and is often described as a saw-toothed pattern. The EOG shows rapid eye movements, while the EMG shows tonic suppression or phasic twitches [30,31]. This EMG activity reflects the two basic components (or divisions) of REM sleep: that is, tonic and phasic. Physiologic phenomena associated with tonic REM sleep include pupillary constriction, widespread skeletal muscle atonia, a decrease in thermoregulation (resulting in decreased body temperature), and the occurrence of sleep-related erections in men and clitoral engorgement in women [58,62]. Phasic REM sleep is marked by rapid eye movements and contraction of the muscles of the middle ear, along with episodes of markedly irregular respiration and heart rate [62].

In the normal young adult, the transition from wakefulness to sleep is through non-REM sleep (usually beginning with Stage 1), with alternating periods of non-REM and REM sleep in cycles that last approximately 90 minutes. Frequent sleep stage changes are common throughout the night, with the composition of stages varying between individuals [51]. While sleep stage patterns are unique to the individual as well as to each specific night, most sleep software constructs a hypnogram to depict the sleep stage changes and progressions that occur during the night that the polysomnogram is recording (Fig. 1). There are hypnograms depicting the generalized sleep stage progression patterns for infancy, childhood, adolescence, and elderly adults, as proportions of sleep stage patterns change across the lifespan [58,63].

Ventilation and sleep

In sleep and wakefulness, the primary purpose of the central respiratory control center is to restrict the fluctuation of arterial blood gas levels to a narrow physiologic range, thus maintaining homeostasis [64]. The three basic types of input that impact ventilatory control are: (1) chemical information regarding pH, arterial partial pressure of oxygen (PaO_2), and $PaCO_2$ from peripheral and central chemoreceptors, (2) mechanical signals from the lung and chest wall (stretch receptors), and (3) behavioral information from the higher centers in the cerebral cortex (ie, wakefulness drive to breathe) [65]. Peripheral chemoreceptors sense decreased levels of PaO_2 and signal the medullary central respiratory control center, resulting in increased ventilation. Elevated levels of $PaCO_2$ are sensed by both the peripheral chemoreceptors and the central chemoreceptors, causing an increase in ventilation via central respiratory control efferent stimulation [65–67]. The wakefulness drive to breathe is absent during sleep; consequently, changes in upper airway mechanics and in central respiratory control occur.

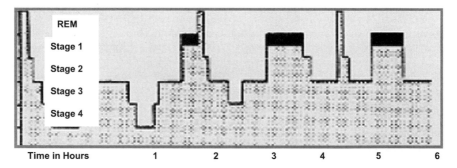

Fig. 1. A hypnogram typical of a young adult. Note the cyclic changes that occur over the course of the sleep time. REM sleep is denoted by the thick black bars. Stages 1 through 4 are depicted as the sleep cycles throughout the night. Most of the slow wave sleep (Stages 3 and 4) occurs at the beginning of the night, while the predominant portion of REM occurs during the latter hours of sleep. In young adulthood, during the first third of the night, slow wave sleep is predominant and is associated with the onset of sleep. REM sleep predominates the last third of the night and is associated with circadian rhythms and body temperature [61]. Non-REM sleep usually constitutes 75% to 80% of the night's sleep, with 5% in Stage 1, 50% in Stage 2, 3% to 8% in Stage 3, and 10% to 15% in Stage 4. REM sleep constitutes 20% to 25% of sleep, while the entire night is usually divided into four to six cycles or episodes [61]. (*Courtesy of* the Respiratory Physiology Laboratory of Jason H. Mateika, PhD, Veterans Administration Medical Center, Detroit, MI; with permission.)

There is a reduction in the caliber of the upper airway during sleep, which is believed to stem from a reduction in upper airway dilating muscle output [68]. This leads to an increase in upper airway resistance [50]. Additionally, there is a lack of load compensation (minute ventilation adjusts to compensate for load) which accounts for a higher level of $PaCO_2$ during sleep [69,70]. There is also an increase in airway compliance and collapsibility during sleep when compared to wakefulness [50]. Cumulatively, the result is a reduced tidal volume and increased $PaCO_2$ that is tolerated for the maintenance of sleep.

Control of upper airway patency

The ability to ventilate is not only dependent on the integrity of medullary respiratory neurons and chest wall muscle contraction, but also on the patency of the upper airway. Of the structures that comprise the upper respiratory tract, the pharynx is the only structure susceptible to collapse [71,72]. Of the 24 pairs of muscles in the upper airway, at least 10 have been categorized as pharyngeal dilator muscles, which operate in a complex and coordinated manner to maintain upper airway patency during wakefulness and sleep [68,73]. Continuous neuromuscular stimulation from medullary cranial motor neurons sustain pharyngeal airway patency during wakefulness [68,72]. Conversely, during sleep there is a reduction in the motoneuron output to the upper airway muscles, resulting in a modest but significant amount of upper airway narrowing [50]. Sleep-related reduction in neural stimulation of the pharyngeal dilator muscles yields little effect on maintenance of airway patency in most individuals. However, in individuals with OSAHS, the balance of pressure within (intraluminal), across (transluminal), and external to the airway (extraluminal) is altered, producing partial or total airway obstruction [47,74]. Apneas and hypopneas are the measurable manifestations of perturbations in these pressures.

Pathophysiology

The causes of pharyngeal collapse in individuals with OSAHS are multifactorial; however, the pharyngeal dilator muscles along with alterations in the central respiratory control center are heavily implicated in the pathogenesis of this disorder [66,67,75,76]. Individuals with OSAHS show a decrease in neuromuscular compensation associated with sleep onset that results in airway narrowing or collapse, with subsequent hypopnea or apnea [57]. $PaCO_2$ increases, while PaO_2 decreases secondary to alveolar hypoventilation. Peripheral and central chemoreceptors are stimulated, resulting in an increase in ventilatory effort. This effort may or may not result in an arousal from sleep, but is sufficient to restore pharyngeal muscle activity such that airway patency is restored. The increase in ventilatory drive during airway patency restoration is associated with initial hyperventilation in an effort to correct derangements in $PaCO_2$ and PaO_2 [77]. Once the airway becomes patent, sleep onset resumes and this scenario repeats cyclically throughout the night (Fig. 2).

When recruitment of the pharyngeal dilator muscles is not sufficient to establish an open airway, then apnea or hypopnea will terminate with an arousal [73]. Arousals are usually brief and often do not result in conscious awakening. The EEG of the polysomnogram will show either a shift to a lighter stage of sleep or a change from sleep to wakefulness [22,58]. While arousals and awakenings are part of normal sleep, individuals suffering from OSAHS and other SDB conditions have an excessive amount (eg, greater than or equal to 20 per hour), resulting in sleep fragmentation [60].

OSAHS and respiratory manifestations

Because apneas, hypopneas, and arousals occur multiple times on an hourly basis throughout the night in individuals with OSAHS, the respiratory neural system that regulates respiratory motor control undergoes mutable changes in response to these perturbations. This demonstrates the presence of neural plasticity in the central respiratory control system [78]. Four intriguing phenomena of recent investigation in the area of OSAHS

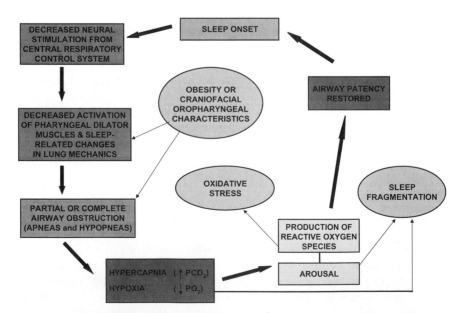

Fig. 2. The cyclical nature of OSAHS. Sleep onset leads to neurologic and physical changes that promote pharyngeal collapse or narrowing in susceptible individuals. Airway occlusion and blood gas alterations lead to arousals, with subsequent production of reactive oxygen species and sleep fragmentation. Once ventilation is resumed, sleep onset recurs and the cycle continues.

are: 1) the hypoxic ventilatory response (HVR), 2) the emergence of a central component in obstructive apnea, 3) long-term facilitation (LTF) of ventilation in individuals with OSAHS, and 4) the presence of oxidative stress. Better understanding of these phenomena is critical to determine whether they individually or collectively promote stability or instability in ventilation during sleep. Knowledge gained regarding these phenomena may uncover insight into the properties of these mechanisms and lead to the development of novel and effective treatment modalities.

Hypoxic ventilatory response

Apnea frequency and severity with OSAHS not only increases during the night, but also over the years, if the individual remains untreated [79–81]. Some hypotheses posited in support of this suggestion are: upper airway muscle fatigue (due to repeated exposure to intermittent hypoxia, resulting in muscle flaccidity); elevation of the arousal threshold throughout the night; and enhancement of the hypoxic ventilatory response (which facilitates an overcompensated response in ventilation, driving the level of $PaCO_2$ below the apneic threshold) [76,82]. The apneic threshold denotes the level of $PaCO_2$ necessary to stimulate breathing by the central respiratory control center during sleep.

Recent studies have shown support for the hypotheses involving the HVR [76,83–85]. An enhancement of peripheral and central chemoreceptor sensitivity stimulates efferent nerve output to increase ventilation and upper airway muscle activity (ie, the phrenic nerve and hypoglossal nerves, respectively) [77,83] and the HVR is the result. This response is the compilation of a multiplicity of independent mechanisms, including but not limited to: the pattern, direction, and intensity of a hypoxic stimulus; the time domain of the stimulus (minutes, weeks, years); effects of the stimulus on breathing (facilitation or depression); effects of the stimulus on the components of breathing (tidal volume, frequency, minute ventilation); and neurotransmitter chemicals inherent to the process (serotonin, dopamine) [84]. Thus, the HVR is present within each individual, yet it has properties of plasticity, whereby the properties can be modified in response to the hypoxic stimulus.

Central component of obstructive apnea

The effect of respiratory neuroplasticity on the HVR is best illustrated in individuals who received tracheostomy as treatment for OSAHS [77,86,87]. Follow-up study in these patients revealed a conversion from obstructive to central apnea, thus unmasking a central respiratory control mechanism present in obstructive apnea [86]. One hypothesis for this central component is that enhancement of the HVR in response to intermittent hypoxia facilitates an overshoot during arousal, subsequently driving the level of $PaCO_2$ below the apneic threshold [67,76,88]. When the $PaCO_2$ is below the apneic threshold during sleep, the drive to breathe is eliminated and apnea ensues until the level of $PaCO_2$ rises sufficiently to stimulate ventilation.

Changes in the HVR may result in increased frequency of apneas throughout the night, shown by the emergence of central apneas during the latter course of sleep [86]. Enhancement of the HVR in the presence of hypocapnea uncovers the apneic threshold, thus perpetuating apnea frequency [66,67,76]. Apnea duration is likewise increased, possibly because of the interaction of hypoxia and hypercarbia resetting the apneic threshold a few millimeters of mercury above or close to the waking ventilatory recruitment threshold [67,77]. The ventilatory recruitment threshold is the point at which $PaCO_2$ drives breathing during wakefulness [66,67,76,85].

Long-term facilitation of ventilation

A third manifestation believed to be inherent to OSAHS is long-term facilitation (LTF) of ventilation. This manifestation of respiratory neuroplasticity was elucidated in humans during wakefulness by Mateika and colleagues [67,76,83,85,88]. LTF is a complex and incompletely understood phenomenon where there is neuromodulated acceleration in ventilation that persists beyond discontinuation of a stimulus, in this case, intermittent hypoxia (a hallmark of OSAHS) [89]. Stimulation of the peripheral and central chemoreceptors after a trial of intermittent hypoxia resulted in a significant increase in ventilatory drive and upper airway muscle activity in healthy individuals. This finding suggests that exposure to intermittent hypoxia during wakefulness leads to increased ventilatory drive secondary to the enhancement of HVR. Harris and colleagues [83] also demonstrated manifestation of LTF after exposure to intermittent hypoxia in individuals with OSAHS. Further studies of LTF in OSAHS during sleep await publication.

Oxidative stress

Oxidative stress has recently been associated with the pattern of events mentioned above, when arterial blood becomes desaturated, followed by hemoglobin resaturation during arousal and restoration of airway patency. More specifically, arousal-related hyperventilation produces a hematologic environment that rapidly changes from low levels of PaO_2 and high levels of $PaCO_2$ to high levels of PaO_2 with low levels of $PaCO_2$. This shift in gas tensions leads to the production and release of reactive oxygen species (ROS), harmful, unstable molecules and anions that are associated with cell damage and destruction [23,25,90,91]. The body's response to ROS production includes release and mobilization of antioxidants from endogenous and exogenous sources, to scavenge free radicals and protect cells from oxidative damage [92,93]. It is postulated that high-level production of ROS results in a significant influx of Ca^{2+} into the cells of the peripheral chemoreceptors. This propagates bursts of neurotransmitter release, resulting in an enhanced peripheral chemoreflex response [89,94]. Hypoxic conditions have also been associated with transient depletion of cellular reductants, which is the basis of antioxidant defense [23,90].

Oxidative stress develops when ROS levels exceed the homeostatic level of antioxidant production and use, causing a shift in balance that favors the oxidative state [25,92]. Studies also suggest that inflammation caused by upper airway collapse and restored patency leads to upper airway mucosal congestion, local inflammation, and oxidative stress [23,90,93,95,96]. The ROS metabolites caused by this phenomenon are present in the tissues, blood, and exhaled breath condensate of individuals with OSAHS. Studies show that individuals with OSAHS have elevated levels of ROS and decreased levels of antioxidants when compared with healthy controls [23,25,90,95].

Cardiovascular manifestations of OSAHS

Hemodynamic alterations

Significant alterations in cardiovascular hemodynamics are evident when comparing normal sleep to the sleep of an individual with OSAHS. In healthy individuals, non-REM sleep comprises 80% of the night, with the cardiovascular system in a state of hemodynamic and sympathetic tranquility (ie, parasympathetic dominance) [97]. During non-REM sleep, blood pressure and heart rate generally show a 10% to15% reduction, with a subsequent 10% decline in cardiac output when compared to wakefulness [98]. REM sleep shows a preponderance of sympathetic activity, whereby heart rate and blood pressure exhibit lability, similar to wakefulness [99]. Conversely, many individuals with OSAHS do not experience the 80% non-REM sleep-related hemodynamic quiescence. Physiologic response to intrathoracic pressure changes related to apnea drives the hemodynamic divergence away from normal sleep via repetitive surges of acute sympathetic activity. Moreover, bursts of sympathetic stimulation during REM sleep are believed to facilitate ventricular dysrhythmias that diminish coronary vascular diastolic filling time [40].

During apnea, pharyngeal collapse leads to a reduction in alveolar oxygen tension (P_AO_2) with subsequent hemoglobin desaturation. Progressive attempts to breathe against a closed or obstructed upper airway renders acute reductions in intrathoracic pressures that may exceed -60 cm H_2O [98]. Greater negative intrathoracic pressure causes an elevation in the transmyocardial pressure gradient, which leads to increased ventricular afterload and augmented venous return, accompanied by a right to left septal shift. Subsequently, there are reductions in left ventricular compliance, left ventricular end diastolic volume, and cardiac output, all of which have further negative implications after resolution of the apnea.

Sympathetic activation

As an apnea progresses toward termination, blood pressure increases steadily, whereas heart rate and cardiac output are reduced. During arousal, surges of sympathetic neural activation increase both heart rate and blood pressure. However, the blood available to oxygenate the myocardium during this time of heightened myocardial demand is desaturated, because the surges of sympathetic activity coincide with the nadir of arterial oxygen desaturation, restoration of ventilation, and arousal from sleep [24,26,100]. Catecholamine levels increase, leading to increased systemic vascular resistance and pulmonary arterial pressures [98]. As these apneic events occur throughout each night and over the years, individuals with OSAHS exhibit a shift toward persistent sympathetic activity during wakefulness, followed by further increases during sleep [15,27]. Individuals typically experience prolonged elevations in heart rate and blood pressure, with a concomitant reduction in vagal activity [52]. Moreover, chronic sympathoadrenal stimulation elevates catecholamine excretion, which intensifies cardiac workload and perpetuates development of cardiac ventricular septal thickness, poor left ventricular diastolic function, endothelial dysfunction, and cardiac rhythm disturbances [27,101].

Vascular endothelial dysfunction

Another cardiovascular manifestation of OSAHS, generating much investigation and debate, is the association between intermittent hypoxia and endothelial dysfunction [16,102,103]. Intermittent hypoxia may mediate the release of potent vasoconstrictors (eg, endothelin-1) as well as suppress release of nitric oxide [102]. Lattimore and colleagues [104] investigated the microvascular endothelium in subjects with OSAHS before and after treatment with CPAP, and found an increase in nitric oxide production and vascular relaxation with the use of CPAP when compared to the baseline state. This suggests endothelial dysfunction may be responsible, in part, for the lack of the circadian blood pressure variability seen in some individuals with OSAHS. Endothelial dysfunction experienced through repetitive apneic events may be a key component in the many chronic vascular diseases associated with OSAHS (eg, atherosclerosis, hypertension, coronary artery disease) [103–105].

Kraiczi and colleagues [105] discovered a dose-dependent relationship between apnea severity (as demonstrated by SaO_2 desaturation) and a slow but significant inclination toward decreased left ventricular diastolic function, along with diminished flow-mediated dilation of brachial arteries. Arterial dilation is largely dependent on generation of nitric oxide from the vascular endothelium. These findings are consistent with a predisposition to atherosclerosis and left ventricular dysfunction. Moreover, these results are especially meaningful because subjects were free from comorbid disease, suggesting a subclinical decline in cardiovascular function before the onset of actual disease.

Inflammatory markers

Inflammation is a key component of many cardiovascular diseases, such as atherosclerosis, ischemic heart disease, and heart failure [99,106]. Increased expression of inflammatory markers has been associated with OSAHS secondary to hypoxemia and sleep deprivation. There is much debate in the literature as to whether certain markers of inflammation have a role in the cardiovascular disease sequelae seen in individuals with OSAHS [26,27,94,99,106,107].

Vascular endothelial growth factor (VEGF) refers to a family of signaling proteins involved in angiogenesis, as well as embryonic vasculogenesis [26]. VEGF production is induced in cells that experience hypoxia. Studies involving high altitude and chronic sustained hypoxia show elevated concentrations of VEGF [108], and several studies have shown significant increases in VEGF that correlate with the degree of nocturnal hypoxia in individuals with OSAHS [108–110]. Moreover, Lavie and colleagues [26] demonstrated a reduction in VEGF following CPAP therapy, and Teramoto and colleagues [111] identified a reduction after a single night of supplemental oxygen administration.

Other critical mediators of inflammatory response and proliferative disorders of the vasculature, such as interleukin (IL-6), C-reactive protein (C-RP), and tumor necrosis factor alpha (TNFα) have also been implicated in the hypoxic response with OSAHS [112]. Vgontzas and colleagues [113] showed reductions in the levels of daytime sleepiness in individuals with OSAHS when given the drug etanercept, a TNFα antagonist. However, these subjects were obese and obesity itself can be considered a proinflammatory state [107]. Direct evidence linking these inflammatory cytokines with pathogenesis of OSAHS is lacking. This is partly because the mechanistic pathway between inflammatory proteins and vascular inflammation that propagates cardiovascular disease involves complex cellular and inflammatory interactions.

Case study

LB was a 26-year-old African American male who responded to an advertisement requesting volunteers for a sleep apnea research study in our laboratory. Study participants included young, healthy, nonobese, nonsmoking individuals with no known medical conditions, who were not taking medications. Participants were self-identified as snorers who wake up with choking sensations or gasping for air, and have had bed partners or family members express concern about their breathing during sleep. LB stated he had not been diagnosed with a sleep disorder and he did not intentionally nap during the day. However, in situations with low environmental stimuli, he was likely to doze. He stated his snoring has been described as "horrible" and that he wakes himself with coughing and choking sensations on a regular basis. His family indicated that he "holds his breath when he sleeps" and his ex-wife expressed a similar concern.

Upon physical examination, LB was a well-developed, well-groomed, well-nourished male, alert and oriented to person, place, and time, and in no apparent distress. He was pleasant and cooperative, maintained good eye contact, and his affect was appropriate to situation; however, he appeared tired. Vital signs included temperature 97.0°(F), pulse 64 beats per minute, respirations 12 per minute, even and nonlabored, and blood pressure 128/56 mmHg. He was 5'9" tall, weighed 185 pounds (body mass index 27.3 kg/m^2), and his neck circumference was 39 cm. Physical assessment was essentially unremarkable except for the oral exam. Only the hard palate was visualized. There was redundant tissue at the base of the tongue, rendering inability to visualize his tonsils or other structures of the soft palate. The uvula was wide and long and rested on the base of the tongue. Mallampati score (which predicts difficult intubation, range 1–4 with 4 indicating maximum difficulty) was class 4. His electrocardiogram exhibited normal sinus rhythm.

During an interview, LB stated that he works in the construction industry and he is saving his money to go to mechanic school, but he has difficulty studying written material as he is likely to fall asleep. He often feels fatigued; however, he pushes himself to work hard. He does not sit down to eat his lunch for fear of falling asleep at work.

LB completed the Epworth Sleepiness Scale (ESS), a global measure of sleep during recent times [114] to quantify his level of daytime sleepiness during the past month. This scale is widely used both in the clinical setting and in sleep research, but is not specific to OSAHS [6,19,115–117]. Scores ranging from 11 to 15 correlate with moderate OSAHS [116]. The ESS is purported to significantly distinguish among subjects with disorders of excessive daytime sleepiness and those without, when correlated with polysomography [118]. LB's total ESS score was 14. He was scheduled for polysomography in our respiratory physiology laboratory. (See Fig. 3 for his sleep hypnogram and Tables 1 and 2 for the results of his study.)

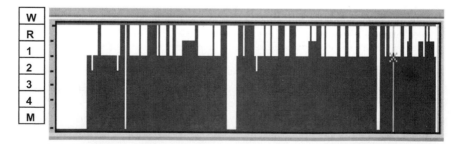

Fig. 3. Sleep hypnogram. Sleep hypnogram for case study LB shows numerous episodes of wakefulness, a predominance of Stage 1 sleep, a small amount of Stage 2 sleep, and three short segments of REM. Note the absence of Stage 3 & 4 (restorative) sleep. W, wake; R, REM; 1, Stage 1; 2, Stage 2; 3, Stage 3; 4, Stage 4; M, movement.

Table 1
Sleep Summary from LB's Polysomnograph Study

Sleep Summary	Minutes	Hours	% (TIB)	% (TST)	% (SPT)
Time in bed (TIB)	553.5	9.2	100.0	N/A	N/A
Total sleep time (TST)	475.0	7.9	85.8	100.0	85.8
Sleep period time (SPT)	553.5	9.2	100.0	N/A	100.0
Total Stage 1 sleep	275.5	4.6	49.8	58.0	49.8
Total Stage 2 sleep	151.0	2.5	27.3	31.8	27.3
Total Stage 3 sleep	0.0	0.0	0.0	0.0	0.0
Total Stage 4 sleep	0.0	0.0	0.0	0.0	0.0
Total REM sleep	48.5	0.8	8.8	10.2	8.8
Total wake time	45.5	0.8	8.2	N/A	8.2
Total movement time	32.5	0.5	5.9	N/A	5.9
Total wake time after sleep onset (SO)	45.5	0.8	8.2	N/A	N/A

LB had 7.9 hours of total sleep time (TST). The remainder of the table shows deviations from normal in the five stages of sleep.

LB exhibited severe obstructive sleep apnea, with 84.9 respiratory-related events per hour of sleep. He experienced approximately 66 apneas per hour and 19 hypopneas, and sleep was extremely disrupted. His lowest oxygen desaturation was 85% during non-REM sleep and 88% during REM sleep. He had no restorative sleep (Stages 3 and 4) during his study. LB was referred for a CPAP titration to reduce or eliminate his apnea.

LB's respiratory manifestations demonstrated an increased HVR, evidenced by the startling number of apneic events per hour. Furthermore, he exhibited a predominance of apneas in relation to hypopneas, suggesting advanced OSAHS. He had central apneas in the latter portion of his polysomnogram, unmasking the central component of OSAHS discussed previously. Evidence of LTF of ventilation could not be ascertained. However, breathing instability was evident by the presence of at least one respiratory event per minute. Cardiovascular manifestations in LB were not apparent however, during his study his heart rate and blood pressure were elevated during and following resolution of his apneic events. During wakefulness, his blood pressure and pulse were typical of a healthy young man. Markers of excessive sympathetic stimulation, endothelial dysfunction, and inflammation were not evaluated. LB has yet to develop outwardly objective cardiovascular sequelae of OSAHS; however, the author cannot state with full

Table 2
AHI Summary from LB's Polysomnograph Study

Apnea Hypopnea Index Summary															
Total A	0.0	0.0	30.3	0.0	30.3	0.0	0.0	66.1	0.0	66.1	0.0	0.0	34.6	0.0	34.6	65.8
Total H	0.0	0.0	1.3	0.0	1.3	0.0	0.0	18.1	0.0	18.1	0.0	0.0	26.0	0.0	26.0	19.1
Total A/H	0.0	0.0	31.6	0.0	31.6	0.0	0.0	84.3	0.0	84.3	0.0	0.0	60.6	0.0	60.6	84.9

LB had an AHI of 84.9 events per hour, 65.8 of the events were apneas and 19.1 of the events were hypopneas. He experienced sleep fragmentation, which may be responsible for his complaint of fatigue, as well as the likelihood of falling asleep during nonstimulating activities.

confidence that the groundwork for cardiovascular disease is not being established.

Implications for nursing

Health-related quality of life has four domains: physical and occupational function, psychological function, social interaction, and somatic sensation [9]. Untreated OSAHS affects well being in each domain due to: daytime sleepiness, difficulty performing tasks requiring sustained attention, impaired social functioning, and fatigue [12,19,49]. Chronically disrupted sleep fraught with arousals makes the problem one that affects the individual 24 hours per day. Individuals suffering from more severe OSAHS demonstrate greater negative impact in these areas [119], thus health related quality of life is reduced as severity of OSAHS increases.

During the years preceding diagnosis, undiagnosed individuals with OSAHS consume twice the medical dollars as healthy individuals. More importantly, medical expenditures decline following the initiation of treatment [120]. Health care costs of individuals with untreated OSAHS also rise proportionately with the presence of comorbid sequelae. In the Sleep Heart Health Study, subjects with mild to moderate sleep disordered breathing (n = 1,023) reported one or more cardiovascular disorders that included myocardial infarction, angina, stroke, heart failure, and need for coronary revascularization procedure [121]. Sleep loss has also been related to poor glycemic control, hyperlipidemia, impaired immune system functioning, and diminished wound healing [122–124]. Clearly, individuals with untreated OSAHS experience multiple respiratory and cardiac manifestations associated with intermittent hypoxia and are at risk for future or further development of pathogenic sequelae that accompany this condition. Thus, health care costs would be greatly reduced if the undiagnosed OSAHS population was identified and appropriately managed.

Screening for sleep disturbance is an important and necessary part of a patient assessment. These evaluations should be conducted by nurses at every level of education and in all health care environments. Patient education interventions focused on the relationship between sleep disruption, fragmentation, and adverse health outcomes are also required for the maintenance of health in patients with OSAHS [7,9].

References

[1] Chung F, Imarengiaye C. Management of sleep apnea in adults. Can J Anesth 2002;49(6): R1–6.
[2] Duran J, Esnaola S, Rubio R, et al. Obstructive sleep apnea-hypopnea and related clinical features in a population-based sample of subjects aged 30 to 70 yr. Am J Respir Crit Care Med 2001;163:685–9.

[3] van Houwelingen KG, van Uffelen R, van Vliet AC. The sleep apnoea syndromes. Eur Heart J 1999;20:858–66.

[4] Kapur V, Blough DK, Sandblom RE, et al. The medical cost of undiagnosed sleep apnea. Sleep 1999;22(6):749–55.

[5] Chervin RD, Murman DL, Malow BA, et al. Cost-utility of three approaches to the diagnosis of sleep apnea: polysomnography, home testing, and empirical therapy. Ann Intern Med 1999;130(6):496–505.

[6] Schlosshan D, Elliott MW. Sleep. 3: Clinical presentation and diagnosis of the obstructive sleep apnoea hypopnoea syndrome. Thorax 2004;59(4):347–52.

[7] Lee KA, Landis C, Chasens ER, et al. Sleep and chronobiology: recommendations for nursing education. Nurs Outlook 2004;52(3):126–33.

[8] Odens ML, Fox CH. Adult sleep apnea syndromes. Am Fam Phys 1995;53(3):859–69.

[9] Moyer CA, Sonnad SS, Garetz SL, et al. Quality of life in obstructive sleep apnea: a systematic review of the literature. Sleep Med 2001;2(6):477–91.

[10] Deegan PC, McNicholas WT. Predictive value of clinical features for the obstructive sleep apnoea syndrome. Eur Respir J 1996;9:117–24.

[11] Young T, Palta M, Dempsey J, et al. The occurrence of sleep-disordered breathing among middle-aged adults. N Engl J Med 1993;328(17):1230–5.

[12] Young T, Peppard PE, Gottlieb DJ. Epidemiology of obstructive sleep apnea: a population health perspective. Am J Respir Crit Care Med 2002;165(9):1217–39.

[13] Caples S, Somers V. Sleep, blood pressure regulation, and hypertension. Sleep Med Clin 2007;2:77–86.

[14] National Heart, Lung, and Blood Institute Working Group on Sleep Apnea. Sleep apnea: is your patient at risk? Am Fam Physician 1996;53(1):247–53.

[15] Gami A, Gregg P, Caples S, et al. Association of atrial fibrillation and obstructive sleep apnea. Circulation 2004;110:364–7.

[16] Krishnan V, Collop N. Sleep and pulmonary hypertension. Sleep Med Clin 2007;2:99–104.

[17] Kaplan J, Staats BA. Obstructive sleep apnea syndrome. Mayo Clin Proc 1990;65(8):1087–94.

[18] Dean RT, Wilcox I. Natural history of sleep apnea, possible atherogenic effects of hypoxia during obstructive sleep apnea. Sleep 1993;16(8):S15–22.

[19] Sleep-related breathing disorders in adults: recommendations for syndrome definition and measurement techniques in clinical research. The Report of an American Academy of Sleep Medicine Task Force. Sleep 1999;22(5):667–89.

[20] Peppard PE, Young T, Palta M, et al. Longitudinal study of moderate weight change and sleep-disordered breathing. JAMA 2000;284(23):3015–21.

[21] Redline S, Strauss ME, Adams N, et al. Neuropsychological function in mild sleep-disordered breathing. Sleep 1997;20(2):160–7.

[22] Redline S, Budhiraja R, Kapur V, et al. The scoring of respiratory events in sleep: reliability and validity. J Clin Sleep Med 2007;3(2):169–200.

[23] Christou K, Moulas AN, Pastaka C, et al. Antioxidant capacity in obstructive sleep apnea patients. Sleep Med 2003;4(3):225–8.

[24] Lavie L, Vishnevsky A, Lavie P. Evidence for lipid peroxidation in obstructive sleep apnea. Sleep 2004;27(1):123–8.

[25] Schulz R, Mahmoudi S, Hattar K, et al. Enhanced release of superoxide from polymorphonuclear neutrophils in obstructive sleep apnea. Impact of continuous positive airway pressure therapy. Am J Respir Crit Care Med 2000;162(2 Pt 1):566–70.

[26] Lavie L. Obstructive sleep apnoea syndrome—an oxidative stress disorder. Sleep Med Rev 2002;7(1):35–51.

[27] Thurnbeer R. Obstructive sleep apnoea and cardiovascular disease—time to act! Swiss Med Weekly 2007;137:217–22.

[28] Aldrich MS. Cardinal manifestations of sleep disorders. In: Kryger M, Roth T, Dement WC, editors. Principles and practice of sleep medicine. 2nd edition. Philadelphia: Saunders; 1994. p. 526–33.

[29] Young T, Skatrud J, Peppard PE. Risk factors for obstructive sleep apnea in adults. JAMA 2004;291(16):2013–6.

[30] Carskadon M, Rechtschaffen A. Monitoring and staging of human sleep. In: Kryger M, Roth T, Dement WC, editors. Principles and practice of sleep medicine. 4th edition. Philadelphia: Elsevier Saunders; 2005. p. 1359–77.

[31] Rechtschaffen A, Kales AA. A manual of standardized terminology, techniques and scoring system for sleep stages of human subjects. Washington, DC: National Institutes of Health; 1968.

[32] Gastaut H, Tassarini C, Duron B. Etudes polygraphiques des manifestations episodiques (hypniques et respiratoires) du syndrome de Pickwick. Rev Neurol 1965;112:568–79 [in French].

[33] Jung R, Kuhlo W. Neurophysiological studies of abnormal night sleep and the Pickwickian syndrome. Prog Brain Res 1965;18:140–59.

[34] Sullivan C, Issa F, Berthon-Jones M, et al. Reversal of obstructive sleep apnoea by continuous positive airway pressure applied through the nares. Lancet 1981;1:862–5.

[35] Caples S, Gami A, Somers V. Obstructive sleep apnea. Ann Intern Med 2005;143(3): 187–97.

[36] Pack A. Advances in sleep-disordered breathing. Am J Respir Crit Care Med 2006;173: 7–15.

[37] Thorpy MJ. Which clinical conditions are responsible for impaired alertness? Sleep Med 2005;1(Suppl 6):S13–20.

[38] Thorpy MJ. Classifications of sleep disorders. In: Kryger M, Roth T, Dement WC, editors. The principles and practice of sleep medicine. 4th edition. Philadelphia: Elsevier Saunders; 2005. p. 615–25.

[39] Berry R, Foster R. Obstructive sleep apnea hypopnea syndromes: Definitions, epidemiology, diagnosis, and consequences. In: Carney P, Berry R, Geyer J, editors. Clinical sleep disorders. Philadelphia: Lippincott Williams & Wilkins; 2005. p. 254–77.

[40] Connolly T, Sharafkhaneh A. Sleep-related breathing disorder and heart disease—central sleep apnea. Sleep Med Clin 2007;2:107–17.

[41] Badr MS. Central sleep apnea syndrome. In: Lee-Chiong TL, Sateia MJ, Carskadon MA, editors. Sleep medicine. Philadelphia: Hanley & Belfus, Inc; 2002.

[42] Schmidt-Nawara W. Obstructive sleep apnea: treatment with oral appliance. Philadelphia: Lippincott Williams & Wilkins; 2005.

[43] Redline S, Kirchner HL, Quan SF, et al. The effects of age, sex, ethnicity, and sleep-disordered breathing on sleep architecture. Arch Intern Med 2004;164:406–18.

[44] Bixler E, Vgontzas A, Lin H-M, et al. Prevalence of sleep-disordered breathing in women, effects of gender. Am J Respir Crit Care Med 2001;163(3Pt1):607–13.

[45] Benumof J. Obstructive sleep apnea in the adult. J Clin Anesth 2001;13:144–56.

[46] Namyslowski G, Scierski W, Mrowka-kata K, et al. Sleep study in patients with overweight and obesity. J Physiol Pharmacol 2005;56(Supp 6):59–65.

[47] Shelton KE, Gay SB, Hollowell DE, et al. Mandible enclosure of upper airway and weight in obstructive sleep apnea. Am Rev Respir Dis 1993;148(1):195–200.

[48] Shelton KE, Woodson H, Gay S, et al. Pharyngeal fat in obstructive sleep apnea. Am Rev Respir Dis 1993;148(2):462–6.

[49] Gottlieb DJ, Yao Q, Redline S, et al. Does snoring predict sleepiness independently of apnea and hypopnea frequency? Am J Respir Crit Care Med 2000;162(4 Pt 1): 1512–7.

[50] Rowley JA, Badr MS. Breathing during sleep: ventilation and the upper airway. In: Carney P, Berry R, Geyer J, editors. Clinical sleep disorders. Philadelphia: Lippincott Williams & Wilkins; 2005. p. 56–72.

[51] Lumb A. Nunn's Applied Respiratory Physiology. 6th edition. Italy: Elsevier; 2005.

[52] Pang K, Terris D. Screening for obstructive sleep apnea: an evidence-based analysis. Am J Otolaryngol 2006;27:112–8.

[53] Jordan AS, McEvoy RD. Gender differences in sleep apnea: epidemiology, clinical presentation and pathogenic mechanisms. Sleep Med Rev 2003;7(5):377–89.

[54] Montoya F, Bedialauneta J, Larrocoechea U, et al. The predictive value of clinical and epidemiological parameters in the identification of patients with obstructive sleep apnoea (OSA): a clinical prediction algorithm in the evaluation of OSA. Eur Arch Otorhinolaryngol 2007;264(6):637–43.

[55] Ferguson KA, Takashi O, Lowe AA, et al. The relationship between obesity and craniofacial structure in obstructive sleep apnea. Chest 1995;108:375–81.

[56] Shellenberg JB, Maislin G, Schwab RJ. Physical findings and the risk for obstructive sleep apnea. Am J Respir Crit Care Med 2000;162:740–8.

[57] Badr MS. Pathophysiology of upper airway obstruction during sleep. Clin Chest Med 1998; 19(1):21–32.

[58] Berry R, Geyer J, Carney P. Introduction to sleep and sleep monitoring—the basics. In: Carney P, Geyer J, Berry R, editors. Clinical sleep disorders. Philadelphia: Lippincott Williams & Wilkins; 2005. p. 3–28.

[59] Fairbanks D. Snoring: A general overview with historical perspectives. In: Fairbanks D, Mickelson S, Woodson B, editors. Snoring and obstructive sleep apnea. 3rd edition. Philadelphia: Lippincott, Williams, Wilkins; 2003. p. 1–17.

[60] Silber M, Krahn L, Morgenthaler T. Sleep Medicine in Clinical Practice. London: Taylor & Francis; 2004.

[61] Carskadon MA, Dement WC. Normal sleep and its variations. In: Kyrger M, Roth T, Dement WC, editors. Principles and practice of sleep medicine. 4th edition. Philadelphia: Elsevier Saunders; 2005. p. 13–23.

[62] Siegel JM. REM sleep. In: Berry R, Roth T, Dement WC, editors. Principles and practice of sleep medicine. Philadelphia: Elsevier Saunders; 2005. p. 120–35.

[63] Ohayon MM, Carskadon MA, Guilleminault C, et al. Meta-analysis of quantitative sleep parameters from childhood to old age in healthy individuals: developing normative sleep values across the human lifespan. Sleep 2004;27(7):1255–73.

[64] West J. Respiratory physiology: the essentials. 6th edition. Philadelphia: Lippincott Williams & Wilkins; 2000.

[65] Douglas N. Respiratory physiology: control of ventilation. In: Kryger M, Roth T, Dement WC, editors. Principles and practice of sleep medicine. 2nd edition. Philadelphia: Saunders; 2005. p. 221–8.

[66] Khodadadeh B, Badr MS, Mateika JH. The ventilatory response to carbon dioxide and sustained hypoxia is enhanced after episodic hypoxia in OSA patients. Respir Physiol Neurobiol 2005;150(2-3):122–34.

[67] Mateika JH, Ellythy M. Chemoreflex control of ventilation is altered during wakefulness in humans with OSA. Respir Physiol Neurobiol 2003;138:45–57.

[68] White DP. Pathogenesis of obstructive and central sleep apnea. Am J Respir Crit Care Med 2005;172(11):1363–70.

[69] Wiegand L, Zwillich C, White DP. Sleep and the ventilatory response to resistive loading in normal men. J Appl Physiol 1988;64:1186–95.

[70] Pillar G, Malhotra A, Fogel R, et al. Airway mechanics and ventilation in response to resistive loading during sleep. Am J Respir Crit Care Med 2000;162:1627–32.

[71] Kuna ST, Remmers JE. Anatomy and physiology of upper airway obstruction. In: Kryger M, Roth T, Dement WC, editors. Principles and practice of sleep medicine. 2nd edition. Philadelphia: Saunders; 1994. p. 838–58.

[72] Qureshi A, Ballard RD. Obstructive sleep apnea. J Allergy Clin Immunol 2003;112(4): 643–51 [quiz: 652].

[73] White DP. Sleep apnea. Proc Am Thorac Soc 2006;3(1):124–8.

[74] Kairaitis K, Stavrinou R, Parikh R, et al. Mandibular advancement decreases pressures in the tissues surrounding the upper airway in rabbits. J Appl Physiol 2006;100(1): 349–56.

[75] Bradford A, McGuire M, O'Halloran KD. Does episodic hypoxia affect upper airway dilator muscle function? Implications for the pathophysiology of obstructive sleep apnoea. Respir Physiol Neurobiol 2005;147(2–3):223–34.

[76] Mateika JH, Mendello C, Obeid D, et al. Peripheral chemoreflex responsiveness is increased at elevated levels of carbon dioxide after episodic hypoxia in awake humans. J Appl Physiol 2004;96(3):1197–205 [discussion: 1196].

[77] Dempsey J, Skatrud J. A sleep-induced apneic threshold and its consequences. Am Rev Respir Dis 1986;133:1163–70.

[78] Dement WC. History of sleep physiology and medicine. In: Kyrger M, Roth T, Dement WC, editors. Principles and practice of sleep medicine. 4th edition. Philadelphia: Elsevier; 2005. p. 1–11.

[79] Charbonneau M, Mairin J, Olha A, et al. Changes in obstructive sleep apnea characteristics through the night. Chest 1994;106:1695–701.

[80] Oksenberg A, Khamaysi I, Silverberg D. Apnoea characteristics across the night in severe obstructive sleep apnoea: influence of body posture. Eur Respir J 2001;18:340–6.

[81] Sforza E, Krieger J, Petiau C. Nocturnal evolution of respiratory effort in obstructive sleep apnoea syndrome: influence on arousal threshold. Eur Respir J 1998;12:1257–63.

[82] Mohan R, Duffin J. The effect of hypoxia on the ventilatory response to carbon dioxide in man. Respir Physiol 1997;108:23–33.

[83] Harris P, Balasubramanian A, Badr MS, et al. Long-term facilitation of ventilation and genioglossus muscle activity is evident in the presence of elevated levels of carbon dioxide in awake humans. Am J Physiol Regul Integr Comp Physiol 2006;291(4):R1111–9.

[84] Powell F, Milsom W, Mitchell G. Time domains of the hypoxic ventilatory response. Respir Physiol 1998;112:123–34.

[85] Ahuja D, Mateika JH, Diamond M, et al. Ventilatory sensitivity to carbon dioxide before and after episodic hypoxia in women treated with testosterone. J Appl Physiol 2007;102: 1832–8.

[86] Fletcher E. Recurrence of sleep apnea syndrome following tracheostomy: A shift from obstructive to central apnea. Chest 1989;96:205–9.

[87] Onal E, Lopata M. Periodic breathing and the pathogenesis of occlusive sleep apneas. Am Rev Respir Dis 1982;126:676–80.

[88] Morelli C, Badr M, Mateika JH. Ventilatory responses to carbon dioxide at low and high levels of oxygen are elevated after episodic hypoxia in men compared with women. J Appl Physiol 2004;97(5):1673–80.

[89] Mitchell G, Johnson S. Plasticity in respiratory motor control. J Appl Physiol 2003;94: 358–74.

[90] Christou K, Markoulis N, Moulas AN, et al. Reactive oxygen metabolites (ROMs) as an index of oxidative stress in obstructive sleep apnea patients. Sleep Breath 2003;7(3): 105–10.

[91] Macey PM, Henderson LA, Macey KE, et al. Brain morphology associated with obstructive sleep apnea. Am J Respir Crit Care Med 2002;166(10):1382–7.

[92] Erel O. A novel automated direct measurement method for total antioxidant capacity using a new generation, more stable ABTS radical cation. Clin Biochem 2004;37(4):277–85.

[93] Row BW, Liu R, Xu W, et al. Intermittent hypoxia is associated with oxidative stress and spatial learning deficits in the rat. Am J Respir Crit Care Med 2003;167(11):1548–53.

[94] Prabhakar N, Dick T, Narduri J, et al. Systemic, cellular and molecular analysis of chemo-reflex-mediated sympathoexcitation by chronic intermittent hypoxia. Exp Physiol 2007; 92(1):39–44.

[95] Carpagnano GE, Kharitonov SA, Resta O, et al. A marker of oxidative stress is increased in exhaled breath condensate of patients with obstructive sleep apnea after night and is reduced by continuous positive airway pressure therapy. Chest 2003;124(4):1386–92.

[96] Ramanathan L, Gozal D, Siegel JM. Antioxidant responses to chronic hypoxia in the rat cerebellum and pons. J Neurochem 2005;93(1):47–52.

[97] Olson L, Svatikova A, Somers VK. Sleep and cardiovascular diseases. In: Carney P, Berry R, Geyer J, editors. Clinical sleep disorders. Philadelphia: Lippincott Williams & Wilkins; 2005. p. 420–34.

[98] Parish J, Somers V. Obstructive sleep apnea and cardiovascular disease. Mayo Clin Proc 2004;79(8):1036–46.

[99] Shamsuzzaman A, Gersh B, Somers VK. Obstructive sleep apnea: Implications for cardiac and vascular disease. JAMA 2003;290(14):1906–14.

[100] Drager L, Pereira A, Barreto-Filho J, et al. Phenotypic characteristics associated with hypertension in patients with obstructive sleep apnea. J Hum Hypertens 2006;20:523–8.

[101] Kaleth A, Chittenden T, Hawkins B, et al. Unique cardiopulmonary exercise test responses in overweight middle-aged adults with obstructive sleep apnea. Sleep Med 2007;8:160–8.

[102] Dincer H, O'Neill W. Deleterious effects of sleep-disordered breathing on the heart and vascular system. Respir 2006;73:124–30.

[103] El Solh A, Akinnusi M, Baddoura F, et al. Endothelial cell apoptosis in obstructive sleep apnea: a link to endothelial dysfunction. Am J Respir Crit Care Med 2007;175: 1186–91.

[104] Lattimore J, Wilcox I, Skilton M, et al. Treatment of obstructive sleep apnoea leads to improved microvascular endothelial function in the systemic circulation. Thorax 2006;61: 491–5.

[105] Kraiczi H, Caidahl K, Samuelsson A, et al. Impairment of vascular endothelial function and left ventricular filling: Association with the severity of apnea-induced hypoxemia during sleep. Chest 2001;119:1085–91.

[106] Ridker P, Buring J, Cook N, et al. C-reactive protein, the metabolic syndrome, and risk of incident cardiovascular events. Circulation 2003;107:391–7.

[107] Phillips C, Yang Q, Williams A, et al. The effect of short-term withdrawal from continuous positive airway pressure therapy on sympathetic activity and markers of vascular inflammation in subjects with obstructive sleep apnoea. J Sleep Res 2007;16:217–25.

[108] Hartman G, Tschop M, Fischer R, et al. High altitude increases circulating interleukin-6, interleukin-1 receptor antagonist and C-reactive protein. Cytokine 2000;12:246–52.

[109] Schulz R, Hummel C, Heinemann S, et al. Serum levels of vascular endothelial growth factor are elevated in patients with obstructive sleep apnea and severe nighttime hypoxia. Am J Respir Crit Care Med 2002;165:67–70.

[110] Zhao Q, Ishibashi M, Hiasa K, et al. Essential role of vascular endothelial growth factor in angiotensin II-induced vascular inflammation and remodeling. Hypertension 2004;44: 264–70.

[111] Teramoto S, Kume H, H Y, et al. Effects of oxygen administration on the circulating vascular endothelial growth factor (VEGF) levels in patients with obstructive sleep apnea syndrome. Intern Med 2003;42:681–5.

[112] Kasabeh E, Chi D, Krishnaswamy G. Inflammatory aspects of sleep apnea and their cardiovascular consequences. South Med J 2006;99(1):58–67.

[113] Vgontzas A, Zoumakis E, Lin H, et al. Marked decrease in sleepiness in patients with sleep apnea by etanercept, a tumor necrosis factor-alpha antagonist. J Clin Endocrinol Metab 2004;89(9):87–91.

[114] Santamaria J. How to evaluate excessive daytime sleepiness in Parkinson's disease. Neurology 2004;63:S21–3.

[115] Fong SYY, Ho CK, Wing YK. Comparing MSLT and ESS in the measurement of excessive daytime sleepiness in obstructive sleep apnoea syndrome. J Psychosom Res 2005;58: 55–60.

[116] Johns M. A new method for measuring daytime sleepiness: the Epworth Sleepiness Scale. Sleep 1991;1(6):540–5.

[117] Petiau C, DKrieger J. Excessive daytime sleepiness. Rev Med Interne 1997;18(3):210–8.

[118] Frank-Stromborg M, Olsen SJ. Instruments for Clinical Health-Care Research. 2nd edition. Sudbury: Jones and Bartlett Publishers; 1997.

[119] Weaver T, George C. Cognition and performance in patients with obstructive sleep apnea. In: Berry R, Roth T, Dement WC, editors. Principles and practice of sleep medicine. Philadelphia: Elsevier Saunders; 2005. p. 1023–33.

[120] Wittmann V, Rodenstein D. Health care costs and the sleep apnea syndrome. Sleep Med Rev 2004;8:269–79.

[121] Shahar E, Whitney CW, Redline S, et al. Sleep-disordered breathing and cardiovascular disease: cross-sectional results of the Sleep Heart Health Study. Am J Respir Crit Care Med 2001;163(1):19–25.

[122] Gottlieb DJ, Punjabi NM, Newman AB, et al. Association of sleep time with diabetes mellitus and impaired glucose tolerance. Arch Intern Med 2005;165(8):863–7.

[123] Gumustekin K, Seven B, Karabulut N, et al. Effects of sleep deprivation, nicotine, and selenium on wound healing in rats. Int J Neurosci 2004;114(11):1433–42.

[124] Schuld A, Haack M, Hinze-Selch D, et al. Experimental studies on the interaction between sleep and the immune system in humans. Psychother Psychosom Med Psychol 2005;55(1):29–35.

ELSEVIER
SAUNDERS

NURSING
CLINICS
OF NORTH AMERICA

Nurs Clin N Am 43 (2008) 77–104

Gender Differences in Knowledge, Attitudes, and Beliefs About Heart Disease

Lynne A. Jensen, PhD, ARNP, BC[a],*,
Debra K. Moser, DNSc, RN, FAAN[b]

[a]Center for the Advancement for Women's Health, College of Nursing, University
of Kentucky, 449 CON Building, 760 Rose Street, Lexington, KY 40536–0232, USA
[b]The Journal of Cardiovascular Nursing, College of Nursing, University of Kentucky,
527 CON Building, 760 Rose Street, Lexington, KY 40536–0232, USA

The purpose of this report is to review the literature on gender differences in knowledge, attitudes, and beliefs about heart disease. Heart disease is the leading cause of death in both men and women in the United States, Europe, and in most developed nations [1]. In the United States alone, approximately 33 million women have a diagnosis of cardiovascular disease (CVD) and more than 500,000 die each year [1]. Despite the significant problem of cardiac disease among women, surveys of women's knowledge, attitudes, and beliefs about the risks of heart disease have continually identified substantial gaps in women's knowledge. For example, in various surveys, only 8% to 46% of women were able to identify heart disease as the leading cause of death in women [2,3]. In a survey of women with known coronary artery disease (CAD), almost half were unaware of their personal risk for heart disease, but many were able to identify that men in their family were at risk for heart disease [4].

The lack of knowledge about heart disease that most women display is of major concern. Although knowledge and appropriate attitudes alone are not sufficient to change behavior, they are necessary to initiate change [5] and spur appropriate action when cardiac symptoms occur. If individuals do not know they are at risk for heart disease, are unable to identify factors that increase their risks for the development of heart disease, or cannot identify signs and symptoms of an acute myocardial infarction (AMI), changes in behavior will not occur [6].

* Corresponding author.
E-mail address: lajens2@email.uky.edu (L.A. Jensen).

0029-6465/08/$ - see front matter © 2008 Elsevier Inc. All rights reserved.
doi:10.1016/j.cnur.2007.10.005   *nursing.theclinics.com*

Although many researchers and clinicians have assumed that women have less knowledge about heart disease than men, these assumptions are based primarily on studies of only women. The few studies in which men and women have been compared suggest that men may be even less knowledgeable than women [7]. Determining whether there are true gender differences in knowledge, attitudes, and beliefs about heart disease is essential so that interventions can be targeted to appropriate groups.

Definitions of knowledge, attitudes, and beliefs

Knowledge, attitudes, and beliefs are independent constructs, but the differences among these constructs are complex, and these constructs were not well differentiated in the literature. These constructs often are used interchangeably to mean the same thing. According to the Cambridge Dictionary [8], knowledge is the understanding of, or information about, a subject that has been obtained by experience or study and is either in a person's mind or possessed by people generally. Attitude is a feeling or opinion about something or someone or a way of behaving that is caused by this attitude or opinion. Belief is the feeling of certainty that something exists or is true. The terms *awareness* and *perception* are often used interchangeably with *knowledge* and *beliefs*. The Cambridge Dictionary [8] defines *awareness* as knowing that something exists or having knowledge or experience of a particular thing. Perception is a belief or opinion often held based on appearances. It has been postulated that cumulative knowledge produces beliefs that when combined with knowledge produce values. These values when combined with social influences produce attitudes [9].

There were no conceptual or operational definitions of knowledge, attitudes, beliefs, or perceptions presented in the heart disease literature reviewed. There was no consensus of what constitutes knowledge, attitudes, or beliefs about heart disease. These terms were used interchangeably in the titles and text of the studies. Given the lack of clarity in the literature reviewed and the classic definitions of the constructs under consideration, in this report, knowledge and awareness were considered as 1 category or construct. Perception and belief were grouped as a second separate category or construct, and attitude was considered a third category.

Data collection

Studies published in the English language on knowledge, attitudes, beliefs, perceptions, and awareness about heart disease were identified by a computerized search of MEDLINE database, PsychINFO, Community of Science, and Cumulative Index to Nursing and Allied Health Literature (CINAHL) between 1990 to present. Multiple subject headings and keyword combinations were used to identify studies for inclusion. Headings (eg, knowledge, attitudes, beliefs, awareness, perceptions, men, and women) were used with heart disease, risks for heart disease, risks for AMI, risks for heart attack, and signs and symptoms of AMI. The reference lists from the original articles were reviewed for any other relevant studies. Many of the studies reviewed reported multiple aspects of heart disease beyond knowledge, attitudes, or beliefs such as sources of information, provider's response to symptoms, and risk-reducing behaviors. For the purposes of this review, only the findings related to knowledge, attitudes, and beliefs were reported.

Results

The studies reviewed are summarized in Table 1.

Knowledge

Knowledge or awareness was considered one category in this discussion.

Knowledge of heart disease as the leading cause of death of women

Studies of women only

There is considerable discrepancy in the literature concerning how well informed women are about heart disease as the leading cause of death in women. In some studies involving only women, knowledge of heart disease as the leading cause of death in women has increased across the last decade from 34% to 46% [3,6]. Yet Prendergast and colleagues [10] in 2004 reported only 13% of their sample was able to identify heart disease as the leading cause of death in women. Despite multiple community campaigns aimed at educating the public about heart disease in women, a majority of women (51% to 55%) were concerned about cancer or breast cancer as their greatest health risk [3,10]. Mosca and colleagues reported that only 40% of women considered themselves well or very well informed about heart disease, but Prendergast and colleagues reported that women rated their knowledge as poor to fair [3,10]. The sample in Prendergast and colleagues' study was 74% African-American compared with 12% in Mosca and colleagues' study, making it difficult to conclude that there are ethnic/racial differences in knowledge. Knowledge level was unrelated to age [3,11]. A majority of younger women, including Hispanics, felt they were less informed about heart disease [3]; however, Wilcox and Stefanick's findings contradict that finding in that younger women were more able to identify heart disease as the leading cause of death in women [6]. In middle-aged women 35 to 44 years of age, only 40% knew that CAD was the leading cause of death in women [3]. Only 34% of women 65 years and older knew that CAD was the leading cause of death [6].

Studies that included both men and women

Few investigators reported findings concerning knowledge about heart disease as the leading cause of death in women. Less than 45% of Europeans

Table 1
Summary of articles on knowledge, attitudes, and beliefs about heart disease

Study	Study type	Sample size	Selected concepts measured	Selected results
Studies of women only				
Pilote and Hlatky [45] Attitudes of women toward hormone therapy and prevention of heart disease	Mailed survey	N = 337 women Median age 50 years	Perceived risk of heart disease	• 73% perceived risk of developing heart disease by age 70 to be 1% • 52% perceived risk of developing breast cancer by age 70 to be ≥10%
Legato et al [35] Women's perceptions of their general health, with special reference to their risk of coronary artery disease: Results of a national telephone survey	Telephone survey, national; 45 questions	N = 1002 women Age 18 + White: 77% AA: 11% Hispanic: 8 %	Women's knowledge of risk for heart disease	• Improvement in health most important concern • 74% knowledgeable about health issues, yet 44% believed somewhat or very unlikely to have AMI • 58% perceived risk of breast cancer same or higher than CAD • 41% of women ≥60 believed women's risk of AMI is lower than male peers
Meischke et al [17] How women label and respond to symptoms of acute myocardial infarction: Responses to hypothetical symptoms scenarios	Telephone survey In Washington State	N = 862 women White: 99% AA: 1%	Hypothetical symptom scenarios; perceived risk of AMI; knowledge of symptoms AMI	• 65% labeled chest pain as AMI symptom • 36% labeled nausea and SOB as AMI symptom • Less than 20% of women who believed their symptoms were AMI would call 911
Wilcox and Stefanick [6] Knowledge and perceived risk of major diseases in middle-aged and older women	In person survey on beliefs and attitudes regarding health and disease; convenience sample	N = 200 women Age: 41–95 White: 86% AA: 5% Hispanic: 4.5% Asian: 2%	Mortality knowledge; perceived general risk; perceived personal risk; knowledge	• 34% older women knew CAD was the leading cause of death among women 65 and older • Women lacked knowledge of leading cause of cancer mortality • Women underestimated personal risk for CAD compared with women's general risk for CAD • Least accurate in belief that women 65 and older are as likely to die from CAD as men 65 and older • Middle-aged and older women lacked knowledge in causes of mortality in women compared with men

Mosca et al [2] Awareness, perception and knowledge of heart disease risk and prevention among women in the US	Telephone survey, national, random; 38-item questionnaire, 4 sections, general awareness of heart disease, communication and behaviors related to CAD prevention, understanding of heart disease in women, demographics	N = 1000 women Age: 25– >65 White: 65% AA: 13% Hispanic: 12.6 %	Awareness of women's health issues; risk factors for CAD; warning signs of AMI	• Majority reported not well informed about heart disease • 20% in each ethnic group were very well informed about heart disease • 51% reported were moderately well informed about heart disease • 31% reported heart disease or stroke leading cause of death • 67% identified chest pain as warning sign • Only 10% were able to identify other warning signs • Only 48% of women >65 were able to correctly state that women are more likely to get heart disease after menopause • 61% stated cancer greatest health risk • Correctly identified heart disease as the leading cause of death in women: White: 33%; AA: 15%; Hispanic: 20%
Oliver-McNeil and Artinian [26] Women's perceptions of personal cardiovascular risk and risk-reducing behaviors	Mailed questionnaire; women with new diagnosis of CAD; mailed questionnaire	N = 33 women Age: 36–85, mean age: 65.64 years White: 100%	Coronary Heart Disease Knowledge Test—used to assess knowledge of risk factors	• Women had limited awareness of personal risk for CAD • Participants' perceptions of risk factors differed from documented risk factors • Mean score of Coronary Heart Disease Knowledge test, 64%
Biswas et al [33] Are women worrying about heart disease?	Mailed questionnaire, Veterans Affairs MC	N = 328 women Age: 36–90, mean age: 49; excluded women with CAD, angina or chest pain White: 77% AA: 33%	Concerns about heart disease; perception of general risk; perception of personal risk	• 42% concerned about heart disease • 84% thought average woman had low lifetime risk of CAD • Older, married women worried less about CAD than younger, unmarried women • Only 46%–59% of women with multiple risk factors were worried about CAD (DM, HTN, smokers)

(continued on next page)

Table 1 (*continued*)

Study	Study type	Sample size	Selected concepts measured	Selected results
King et al [34] Perception of risk for coronary heart disease in women undergoing coronary angiography	Face to face interview of women undergoing coronary angioplasty	N = 450 women Age: 32–92 Mean: 64.5 White: 94% AA: 5.8% Hispanic: 0.2%	Perception of CAD risk	• 35% women recalled being told they were at risk for CAD even though 84% had 3 or more risk factors • Younger, more educated women more likely to remember were told at risk for CAD
Marcuccio et al [4] A survey of attitudes and experiences of women with heart disease	Telephone survey; women self- reported diagnosis of CAD or other cardiac diseases	N = 204 women Age: 20–80s; 52% between 40–59	Knowledge and attitudes about heart disease	• 45% did not know they were at risk for CAD • 62% reported had a family history that put them at risk for CAD • 55% had a high level of awareness of personal cardiac risk • 36% recognized initial symptoms as cardiac in origin • Heart disease a "man's" disease • Advice: "Educate yourself and ask questions"
Mosca et al [3] Tracking women's awareness of heart disease An American Heart Association national study	National telephone survey	N = 1024 women Age 25–>65 White: 68% AA: 12% Hispanic: 12% Other: 8%	Awareness, knowledge and perception of CVD risk; risk factors and perceptions of CVD	• 51% stated cancer greatest health risk (35% breast cancer greatest health risk, 16% cancer in general) • 40% considered themselves well informed about heart disease • 13% cite heart disease as their greatest health problem • 46% identified heart disease as the leading cause of death in women (increased from 30% in 1997) • 40% well or very well informed about heart disease • 89% recognize early treatment exists for AMI • Minority of women able to identify risk factors of CAD

Study	Method	Focus	Findings
Prendergast et al [10] Knowledge of heart disease among women in an urban emergency setting	Face-to-face survey of women presenting to emergency room	N = 200 women Age: 25–44 74% AA	Greatest health risk for women; knowledge of risk factors for heart disease; symptoms of AMI	• 13% women correctly identified heart disease as leading cause of death in women • 6% felt heart disease greatest health issue for women • 55% felt breast cancer greatest health risk • Half of the women were able to identify 3 traditional risk factors: hypercholesterolemia, hypertension, tobacco • Majority of women rated knowledge of heart disease as fair to poor • Almost half indicated little-to- no knowledge of AMI symptoms • 87% identified chest pain as symptoms of AMI • Less than 1/3 were familiar with atypical symptoms of AMI
Wyatt and Ratner [15] Evaluating treatment – seeking for acute myocardial infarction in women (Canada)	Telephone survey, questionnaire	N = 349 women Age: 18 –91 Mean age: 47	Symptoms of AMI, susceptibility to AMI; general risk factors for AMI; response to symptoms of AMI	• 23% stated women not at all likely to have AMI compared with men • 55% stated it was possible that women may have AMI • 12% considered their risk for AMI as likely • 8.3% considered their risk for AMI as very likely • 75% indicated a need to better recognize symptoms of AMI • If had symptoms longer than 10 minutes, call hospital or ambulance, more than 50% would go to the hospital or call ambulance

(continued on next page)

Table 1 (*continued*)

Study	Study type	Sample size	Selected concepts measured	Selected results
Studies of men and women				
Shepherd et al [13] International comparison of awareness and attitudes toward coronary risk factor reduction: the HELP study	Interview of public and individual at risk for CAD	N = 10,018 Women = 5006 Men = 5024 Men aged 40–69 Women aged 50–69 Four groups: general public, high-risk public, post- MI patients, post-MI relatives	Awareness and attitudes to coronary heart disease; frequency of health-related behaviors practiced	• Low level of worry about heart disease by general public and high-risk group • Cancer was the most important health concern • Heart disease and cancer were cited as the leading causes of death
Johnson and King [21] Influence of expectations about symptoms on delay in seeking treatment during a myocardial infarction	Questionnaire, semi-structured interview retrospective, descriptive; patients after AMI	N = 65 Women: 17 Men: 48 Age range: 29–85; mean 57.2 ± 12.7 White: 86%	Symptom Representation questionnaire – expectations about heart disease	• 83% expected pain • 47% expected associated symptoms —SOB, perspiration, dizziness • Expectations did not match experience for 74% of subjects
Zerwic et al [30] Perceptions of patients with cardiovascular disease about the causes of coronary artery disease	Interview- Qualitative study of patients with new diagnosis of CAD	N = 105; 65 with acute AMI 53 evaluated for CAD by angiography Women: 34 Men: 71 Mean age: +57.2 ± 12.7 (29–85) White: 86 % AA: 11% Hispanic: 1.5%	Perception about risk factors as causes of CAD; Personal perception of cause of CAD	• Most frequently cited cause of CAD were diet and smoking • 19% MI patients and 40% angioplasty patients were not sure of personal cause of CAD

Zerwic [19] Symptoms of acute myocardial infarction: Expectations of a community sample	Street-intercept survey (urban setting)	N = 414 Women: 197 Men: 217 Age: 19–82 Mean age: 41 White: 40% AA: 29.2% Hispanic: 20% Asian: 9.7%	Representation of Heart Attack Symptom questionnaire—expectations of AMI symptoms	• 99.8% expected chest pain with AMI • 97% expected palpitations and irregular heart beats with AMI • 77%–93% expected discomfort of AMI to be severe • 84% women compared with 73% men expected discomfort in left shoulder • No ethnic differences in identification of symptoms of AMI • Gender differences: women expected discomfort in left shoulder and left arm more then men • Women also expected shills with AMI more than men
Van Tiel et al [29] Sex differences in illness beliefs and illness behavior in patients with suspected coronary artery disease	Interview of patients with suspected CAD	N = 28 Women: 16 Men: 12 Mean age women: 58 Mean age men: 63	Estimate probability of developing CAD in men, women and themselves; lifetime probability of CAD, knowledge of risk factors	• Women estimate own lifetime probability of CAD at 30% (actual 41%) • Men estimate own lifetime probability of CAD at 32% (actual 66%) • Both men and women think of CAD as a "mans disease" • Men and women equally well informed about risk factors—able to identify 2.3 risk factors • Most men and women did not attribute symptoms to heart when seeking medical care; no gender differences noted • Women waited longer to contact primary care physician provider for symptoms

(continued on next page)

Table 1 (*continued*)

Study	Study type	Sample size	Selected concepts measured	Selected results
Kirkland et al [27] Knowledge and awareness of risk factors for cardiovascular disease among Canadians 55 to 74 years of age: results of the Canadian Heart Health Survey, 1986–1992 (abstract)	Home interview; descriptive, cross-sectional survey	N = 4976	Knowledge and awareness of CAD risk factors	• Smoking or stress major causes of heart disease (41% and 44%) • Women more aware than men that hypertension and heredity were risks for CAD • Women smokers were more aware of risk factors than men • Women with AMI were more aware than men of major causes of AMI • Awareness of risk factors lower in older age group • 62% men and 67% women unaware of cholesterol status
Ayanian and Cleary [38] Perceived risks of heart disease and cancer among cigarette smokers	Telephone and self-administered survey of US households; 3 groups: current smoker, former smoker, nonsmoker	N = 3031 Women = 1016 Men = 1317 M = 38%–50% Mean age: 42–49 White: 80%–84% AA: 9.6%–12.8%	Risk of AMI higher, lower or same as men/woman your age	• Smokers: 29% perceived risk of AMI • Heavy smokers (>40/day) 39% perceived risk for AMI • Former smokers: 15% perceived risk for AMI • Non-smoker: 15% perceived risk for AMI
Goff et al [20] Knowledge of heart attack symptoms in a population survey in the united states	Random-digit dialed telephone questionnaire	N = 1294 Women: 735 Men: 547 Age: 18–>55 White: 75% AA: 8.2% Hispanic: 11.2%	Knowledge of symptoms of AMI	• 89.7% identified chest pain as a heart attack symptom • More than 50% identified pain as the most important symptom • Less knowledge of risk factors in oldest group, >55 • Risk factor status not associated with knowledge of heart attack symptoms • Previous experience with CAD, either personal, family, or friend, all more knowledgeable about complex presentation of AMI • Greater level of knowledge of risk factors in whites than other ethnic groups; in 35–55 age group, more educated and higher income groups

Source	Method	Sample	Variables	Findings
Meischke et al [11] Factors that influence personal perceptions of the risk of an acute myocardial infarction	Random-dialed survey—part of REACT trial	N = 1294 Women: 738 Men: 456 Age: 18–>55 White: 75% AA: 8.2% Hispanic: 11.2%	Perceived risk of AMI; Knowledge of AMI; Heart disease most common cause of death in women in USA	• 45% somewhat or less likely to have AMI in 5 years • 31% knew heart disease most common cause of death in women • 75% stated most AMIs occur in people over age 65 • 75% rated AMI risk the same or less likely than people same age • Gender, age, race, and education were not associated with risk perception
Finnegan et al [22] Patient delay in seeking care for heart attack symptoms; findings from focus groups in 5 US regions	Focus groups with adults with previous AMI, high risk for AMI	N = 34 focus groups of 207 participants (did not report number of women or men) Adults > 30	Symptom expectation/experiences; symptom attribution; personal risk perception; knowledge of benefits; barriers	• 8 of 10 during first event did not believe symptoms were AMI • Women have lower personal risk; CAD a "male problem" • Women attributed symptoms to other chronic conditions • Women did not understand increased risk for AMI after menopause • Minority of women waited longer to seek care • Both men and women had little knowledge of reperfusion • Men stated they were "too young" to experience an AMI
Murray [43] The interplay between social and cultural context and perceptions of cardiovascular disease	Qualitative study with post-AMI patients; 3 questionnaires	N = 10 patients, 10 significant other, 10 staff Age: 31–74 years; mean age: 61	Perceptions of patients' cardiovascular risk	• Perception of cardiovascular risk factors: work related, stress, and fate most common risk factors • Fate played part in patient's illness

(continued on next page)

Table 1 (*continued*)

Study	Study type	Sample size	Selected concepts measured	Selected results
Andersson and Leppert [7] Men of low socio-economic and educational level possess pronounced deficient knowledge about the risk factors related to coronary heart disease (Sweden)	Interview at health care center	N = 1011 Women: 554 Men: 457 Age: 50	Knowledge of CHD risk factors (attention given to educational and socio-economic status)	• Women were more knowledgeable than men about risk factors for CHD independent of education or socio-economic status • Low education and low socio-economic status related to poor knowledge of risk factors • Majority reported deficient knowledge of CAD risk factors
Pattenden et al [5] Decision making processes in people with symptoms of an acute myocardial infarction: qualitative study	Qualitative study; patients with known CAD—post-AMI	N = 22 Women: 2 Men: 20 Mean age: 66	Perceived risk of AMI	• Many did not perceive themselves at risk—delayed longer • People with previous CABG or angioplasty believed they were no longer at risk for AMI—delayed longer • 35% women and 68% physicians correctly recognized symptoms as potentially related to the heart
Erhardt and Hobbs [12] Public perception of cardiovascular risk in five European countries: the react survey (abstract)	Face-to-face interviews	N = 5104 Women = 2611 Men = 2493	Attitudes and behaviors: general and personal risk factors for CHD	• 45% public correctly identified CHD as the leading cause of death in their country • 51% aware that high cholesterol increased CHD risk • Swedes and Germans most aware of CHD risk factors
King [32] Illness attributions and myocardial infarction: the influence of gender and socio-economic circumstances on illness beliefs	Phenomenology—interviews of individuals diagnosed with AMI admitted to hospital	N = 24 Women = 12 Men = 12	Perceptions of cause of myocardial infarction	• Stress was cited as the most common cause of their illness • Men also cited behavioral or lifestyle factors in illness onset

Study	Method	Sample	Focus	Findings
Frijling et al [37] Perceptions of CVD risk among patients with hypertension of diabetes (The Netherlands)	Questionnaires mailed to patients with hypertension and diabetes in general practice	N = 1557 Women: 903 Men: 654 Mean age: 62.5 years	Perception of risk for CAD; estimate of 10 year risk for AMI	• 80% self-rated health good to excellent • 50% overestimate risk for CAD • Men more accurate in risk for CAD
McDermott et al [40] Knowledge and attitudes regarding cardiovascular disease risk and prevention in patients with coronary or peripheral arterial disease	Interview of patients in 3 groups: patients with no disease, PAD, CAD	N = 348 Men = (3 groups) 65; 72; 42 Women = (3 groups) 77; 64; 28 Mean age: 68–70.8 years AA: 15% –25%	Perceptions of risks of CAD in patients with known CAD or PAD – given hypothetical patient with CAD or PAD	• Patients with PAD did not see themselves at risk for AMI, stroke, or death • 70% of all 3 groups believed risk for AMI extremely high for patient with CAD • 23% believed patient with PAD at risk for AMI
Montgomery et al [41] Family and friends with disease: their impact on perceived risk	Questionnaire	N = 522 Women: 323 Men: 198 Mean age: 18 years and older; mean age: 40 White: 56% AA: 15% Hispanic: 12%	Perceived risk, personal and family history; non-family, or friends with a history of diseases	• Women with family and friend history increased perceived risks • Men with only family history increased perceived risks • Age, education, marital status, and ethnicity were not associated with perceived risks of heart disease
Green et al [28] Heart disease risk perception in college men and women	Questionnaire distributed in selected classes	N = 470 Women = 255 Men = 215 Mean age: 22.2 years White: 86% AA: 5.5% Hispanic: 6.4%	General perceptions of heart diseases risks; perceptions of strength of causality of CHD risk markers and AMI	• 68% believed risk for AMI lower than peers • Significant number did not understand basic causal relationships in the development of CAD • No gender differences in perception of overall cardiac risk

(continued on next page)

Table 1 (*continued*)

Study	Study type	Sample size	Selected concepts measured	Selected results
Ferrario et al [39] People's perception of their overall coronary risk: an Italian experience	Questionnaire	N = 887 Women: 495 Men: 382 Mean age: 57.9 years Range: 32–>80	Perception of coronary risk – assess own overall risk for coronary risk in next 10 years	• 56% estimated low/mild risk for CAD • 9% high/very high risk • 40% overestimated risk • 27% underestimated risk • Men, ≥65, history of DM, and low educational level underestimate risk for CHD • DM, older age, and male not considered important risk factors • Persons with high coronary risk are unaware of risk and causal factors
Momtahan et al [25] Patients' understanding of cardiac risk factors: A point-prevalence study	Interview— hospitalized patients; 3 parts to interview— patient, significant other, and chart	N = 71 Women: 27 Men: 44 Age: 18 to 74 years N = 53 significant others	Understanding of cardiac risk factors in general, personal cardiac risk factors	• Most patients unable to define cardiac risk factor spontaneously, but given multiple choices, almost all identified correctly • Average general knowledge score 13.6/16 of cardiac risk factors; not statistically different between men and women • Patients identified on average 6 personal risk factors (0–13)
Collins et al [14] Heart disease awareness among college students	Questionnaire distributed in selected classes	N = 1420 Women: 805 Men: 615 White: 75.1% AA: 7.3% Hispanic: 12.5%	Knowledge of heart disease risk factors; perceptions of own health risks	• Overall, 44% believed cancer was greatest risk • 49% women versus 37% men believed cancer was greatest risk • Overall, 24% believed heart disease greatest risk • Overall, 69% believed heart disease most significant cause of death in men • Overall, 67% believed cancer is number one cause of death in women

Greenlund et al [18] Public recognition of major signs and symptoms of heart attack: Seventeen states and the US Virgin Islands, 2001	Telephone survey Questionnaire	N = 61,081 Women: 36,087 Men: 24,931 Age: 18 – >80 White: 79.7% AA: 10.2% Hispanic: 3.9%	Recognition of symptoms of AMI; Response to symptoms AMI	• 92% correctly recognized ≥3 symptoms of AMI • 95% recognized chest pain or discomfort as symptoms of AMI • 86% indicated they would call 911 when they thought someone was having a heart attack • Only gender difference, men less likely to classify jaw pain as symptom of AMI • 11% of persons recognized major symptoms of AMI and knew to call 911 • Whites somewhat more knowledgeable than other ethnic groups to know symptoms of AMI
Tullmann and Dracup [23] Knowledge of heart attack symptoms in older men and women at risk for acute myocardial infarction	Face-to-face survey: Response questionnaire	N = 115 Women = 60 Men = 55 Age: ≥65 White: 72.1% Hispanic: 12.1% AA: 6.9%	Knowledge of AMI symptoms	• ≥95% of men and women recognized chest pain, pressure or tightness, arm or shoulder pain, sweating, and shortness of breath as common symptoms of AMI • 50%–70% of men and women know less common symptoms of AMI: neck pain, nausea, vomiting back pain, jaw pain, heartburn, malaise • 60% of women compared with 40% of men knew jaw pain was a symptom • 62% of men and only 42% of women knew headache was not a symptom of AMI

Abbreviations: AA, African American DM, diabetes mellitus; HTN, hypertension; PAD, peripheral arterial disease; SOB, shortness of breath.

identified CAD as the leading cause of death in their country [12,13]. There were no questions as to the leading cause of death in men versus women, and there was no comparison of responses by gender. In college-age men and women, 69% believed that heart disease was the most significant cause of death in men, and 67% believed cancer was the number one killer of women [14].

Knowledge of heart disease as the leading cause of death was suboptimal in women and men and appeared to be unrelated to age. There were too few studies in which racial/ethnic differences were investigated to draw any conclusions about the impact of racial/ethnic differences on knowledge of heart disease.

Knowledge of symptoms of acute myocardial infarction

The study of people's knowledge of AMI symptoms has been hindered by methodologic problems. The major problem has been the failure to use reliable and valid measurements of symptoms. The psychometric properties of these instruments have seldom been reported. The list of symptoms of an AMI varied among the studies. Decoy symptoms often were included in many of the questionnaires to control for acquiescence in responding to all symptoms listed.

Studies of women only

In studies of women only, 62% to 87% thought that chest pain was the most common symptom presentation of an AMI [2,3,10,15,16], and they expected the pain to be severe [15]. Only 10% to 40% of the women were able to identify less common or less well known symptoms of an AMI such as dizziness, diaphoresis, shortness of breath, nausea, and fatigue [2,3,10,17]. Wyatt and Ratner reported that 57% of the women felt that women would experience the same symptoms of an AMI as men [15]. More than 75% of women indicated they needed a better understanding of the symptoms of an AMI to identify symptoms in themselves [15]. Almost 50% of a sample of African-American women had little to no knowledge of symptoms of an AMI, and less than one third were familiar with less well known symptoms of AMI [10]. These findings raise the question of whether there are ethnic differences in knowledge of AMI symptoms.

Studies that included both men and women

In studies of both men and women, chest pain was the most commonly recognized symptom of an AMI [6,10,17–21], and 77% to 93% of men and women expected the pain of a heart attack to be severe [15,19,21]. The expectation of severe pain may be promoted by media images of AMI of the so-called "Hollywood" heart attack [22]. Such "Hollywood" heart attacks are not the common experience.

Johnson and King [21] reported that 74% of subjects who had an AMI reported experiencing symptoms that did not match their expectations.

Symptoms expected included shortness of breath, vomiting, diarrhea, light-headedness, and blurred vision [20,21].

Atypical or uncommon symptoms of an AMI, such as neck pain, jaw pain, and back pain were more frequently recognized by women than men [18,19]. Greenlund and colleagues [18] reported that 92% of study participants correctly recognized three or more symptoms of an AMI, but only 11% correctly identified all symptoms.

Men and women aged 65 and older were less knowledgeable about symptoms of an AMI than younger adults [23], but individuals with a previous experience with CAD were more knowledgeable about symptoms than those without CAD [24]. Zerwic [19] found no ethnic differences in the ability of women to identify symptoms of AMI. Goff and colleagues [20] reported no gender differences in knowledge, but a higher socioeconomic status and higher education level was associated with higher knowledge of symptoms of an AMI.

Both men and women identified chest pain as the most common symptom of AMI, but the atypical or less well known AMI symptoms were more often recognized by women than men [18,19]. Higher education and socioeconomic levels were associated with more knowledge concerning symptoms of AMI [20]. Men and women older than 65 years were less knowledgeable about symptoms of AMI [23,24].

Knowledge of risk factors for AMI

Correct identification of risk factors depends on whether participants have to recall risk factors [3,25] from memory or recognize risk factors from a list provided [7,10,26]. There was no consensus among the studies concerning the risk factors included in the questionnaires. In addition to tobacco, hypertension, hyperlipidemia, diabetes, and obesity, some studies included menopause, either natural or surgical, decreased estrogen [26], and second hand smoke as risk factors. Physical activity and stress were also considered risk factors for AMI in some studies [7,10,25]. Knowledge scores were reported in a few studies, but there was no consistent tool used to evaluate knowledge of heart disease or risk factors.

Studies of women only

Smoking, high cholesterol, high blood pressure, obesity, and stress were the risk factors most commonly identified by women [10,15]. Mosca and colleagues [3] and Prendergast and colleagues [10] reported ethnic/racial differences in identification of risk factors but the unequal racial composition of these samples raises questions about conclusions that can be drawn from their results. Mosca and associates [3] also found that in women 35–64 years of age, white women were more likely to correctly identify major risk factors than women in other racial/ethnic groups. Few women in any racial/ethnic group were able to correctly identify risk factors for CAD and few women with CAD could identify their own risk factors [3]. Oliver-McNeil and Artinian found no significant relationship between education level or age and knowledge of risk factors [26].

Studies that included both men and women

Smoking, diet, obesity, high blood pressure and stress were the cardiac risk factors identified most commonly by male and female study participants [7,12,25,27,28]. In a group of hospitalized patients, Momtahan and colleagues found the overall general risk factor knowledge score for AMI was 13.5 out of a possible 16. No gender differences in mean scores were identified, but a higher level of education was associated with a higher knowledge score [7,25]. No gender differences in knowledge were found in Van Tiel and colleagues' study [29]. In contrast, in Andersson and Leppert's study of 50-year-old men and women, women had better knowledge of CAD risk factors than men, but the majority of participants felt they lacked knowledge about CAD [7]. Low socioeconomic status and lower educational level also influenced knowledge levels [7]. In Zerwic and colleagues' study of high risk individuals, 79% could name one cardiac risk factor, but only 7% could name three risk factors [30].

In a group of men and women who presented to their general practitioner with chest pain, there were no gender differences in ability to recognize risk factors [29]. In a Canadian study, women were more knowledgeable than men in identifying risk factors but awareness of risk factors was lower in the older age group (65-74 years) [27]. College age men and women believed high blood pressure was the greatest risk factor for CAD, followed by heredity, smoking and stress [14].

In summary, there was no consensus regarding factors that influenced or predicted knowledge of risk factors for CAD, but higher education and socioeconomic status were associated with better knowledge scores [7,25]. Knowledge of CAD risk factors was limited in both men and women.

Attitudes toward seeking care for symptoms of AMI

Studies of women only

Women who had undergone coronary artery bypass graft (CABG) surgery or percutaneous coronary intervention (PCI) delayed seeking care for symptoms of AMI because they no longer perceived themselves to be at risk for CAD, and they did not seek care until symptoms became unbearable [5]. Yet, when women were asked if they or someone they knew was experiencing symptoms of a heart attack, 93% agreed the most important thing to do was get to the hospital, and 86% said the most important thing to do was to call 911 [16].

Wyatt and Ratner reported 35% of women surveyed wanted to be sure they were having a heart attack before going to the emergency department, and more women chose to go to the emergency room by their own means rather than call 911 [15]. Meischke and colleagues found that only 20% of women surveyed would call 911 in response to symptoms of AMI [17].

Studies that included both men and women

Van Tiel and colleagues reported that most men and women who sought medical care for an event did not attribute the symptoms they were experiencing to the heart [29]. Almost 80% of men and women did not believe that the symptoms they experienced at the time of an AMI were related to a heart attack [22]. Yet, 50% to 90% of individuals say they would act quickly in response to symptoms of an AMI and call 911 [15,16,18]. Greenlund and colleagues reported that only 11% of their sample knew all the symptoms of an AMI and would call 911 if someone were having symptoms of a heart attack. Women often delayed seeking care because they did not perceive themselves to be at risk for AMI and thought heart disease was primarily a man's disease [22,29].

Finnegan and colleagues reported that neither men nor women planned what they would do in the event of an AMI, nor did they discuss a plan with their health care provider [22]. The majority of men and women were with others when symptoms of AMI occurred. Most discussed their symptoms with spouses, coworkers, or friends who encouraged the individual to seek care. Many individuals delayed seeking care until their symptoms worsened. African-American and Hispanic women delayed longer than other groups [22]. Women were more dissatisfied than men with their health care provider when discussing their symptoms and actions in response to AMI symptoms [22].

There appear to be few gender differences in attitudes toward seeking care for cardiac symptoms. Although individuals in most studies indicated they would respond quickly and appropriately, current research indicates most individuals delay in seeking care for symptoms of AMI [31].

Beliefs

Belief and perceptions were considered as 1 category in the following discussion.

Beliefs about risks for coronary artery disease/acute myocardial infarction

Studies of women only. Most women, especially older women, did not see themselves at risk for CAD despite having risk factors or health problems that put them at risk [32]. Less than 42% of healthy women were concerned about heart disease, although this proportion increased to 59% when women had up to 3 CAD risk factors [33]. In a group of women with known risk factors for CAD, only 35% of the sample remembered being told they were at risk for CAD at the time of angioplasty [34].

Biswas and colleagues [33] reported that older, married women worried less than younger, unmarried women did, but 84% thought the average woman had a low lifetime risk of CAD. Legato and colleagues reported that 44% of the women in their study believed that it was somewhat or very unlikely that they would have a heart attack, and 41% of older women did not perceive themselves to be at risk [35]. These women also believed that women over 60 were at lower risk for AMI than their male counterparts [35].

In a Canadian study, only 12% of women considered themselves to be at risk for an AMI; only 8.3% of the women surveyed considered themselves very likely to have an AMI [15]. Women who had undergone either PCI or CABG surgery believed they were no longer at risk for CAD and were unsure how to respond to recurrence of symptoms after the procedures [5].

Finnegan and colleagues reported that the majority of women believed that CAD/AMI was a man's disease and that more than 50% were surprised when they had a heart attack [22]. Older women did not recognize their increased risk for CAD; they thought their risk was caused by other health problems [22].

Studies that included both men and women. Findings from the Rapid Early Action for Coronary Treatment (REACT) study showed that only 21% of men and women in the sample believed they were somewhat or more likely than other people their age to have an AMI [36]. Personal perceptions of risk for AMI increased with age and poorer general health [11]. This is in contrast with Meischke and colleagues' findings in 2002, in which 72% of women felt that during their lifetime they were somewhat or very likely to have a heart attack. Older age, smoking, family history, and perceived poor health predicted higher levels of perceived risk for CAD in a high-risk population [37]. Thirty-nine percent of heavy smokers believed they had a higher-than-average risk for AMI [38]. Approximately 50% of women with known heart disease knew they were at risk for CAD, but 45% of the women felt the diagnosis of CAD was a complete surprise [4].

When people were asked to estimate their risk for CAD/AMI, both women and men tended to underestimate their risks [6,29]. Women estimated their risk at 30% (actual risk 41%) and men estimated their risk at 32% (actual risk 66%) [29]. Only 35% of women undergoing coronary angiography remembered ever having been told they were at risk for CAD [34]. Having a history of diabetes, being male, having a lower educational level, and being over 65 years was associated with underestimating risk for CAD [39]. In contrast, Frijling and colleagues [37] found that individuals with hypertension or diabetes tended to overestimate their risk for CAD. Among smokers, only 29% perceived themselves to be at risk for AMI [38]. Smoking increases a person's risk of dying from CAD by 2- to 3-fold and was responsible for more than 125,000 cardiac deaths [1].

McDermott and colleagues [40] asked a group of high-risk individuals with known CAD or peripheral arterial disease (PAD) and a group without CAD to estimate their risks for AMI. Almost 70% of the individuals with PAD, a group at high risk for AMI, believed an individual with CAD was at very high risk for AMI, but only 13% of these high-risk individuals believed an individual with PAD was at risk for AMI [40]. In the group of individuals with CAD, 70% estimated the risk for an AMI to be extremely high, but only 13%

of the group thought an individual with PAD was at risk for an AMI [40]. Even though individuals with PAD are at high risk for CAD, these individuals did not make the connection between CAD and PAD.

Having a family member or friend with heart disease can influence an individual's perception of their risk for AMI. Women having family or a friend with CAD expressed increased perception of their own risk [4]. Family history, but not friends with CAD, influenced men's perception of their risk for CAD [41]. In another study, women with a family history of CAD had a higher perception of risk for CAD [42].

In contrast to an older population, college-age men and women underestimated their risk for CAD [14,28]. Most of the students did not understand the relationship between risk factors and the development of CAD [14]. In a study of African-Americans and Hispanics, both high-risk groups, participants believed that whites were most affected by CAD [10].

Both men and women failed to see themselves at risk for CAD and, when asked, underestimated their risks [6,11,29]. Family history positively influenced perceptions of both men and women [42]. Most older men and women did not believe they were at risk for CAD [33,37,39].

Beliefs about cause of coronary artery disease/acute myocardial infarction

When asked about the causes of a heart attack, many factors were identified. Work, stress, fate, smoking, and diet as well as traditional risk factors for heart disease were stated as potential causes of CAD/AMI [3,27,30,43].

Studies of women only
Less than one third of women were able to identify the major risk factors that cause heart disease [3]. Poor dietary habits and stress were also reported as perceived causes of heart disease [3,30].

Studies that included both men and women
Both men and women believed smoking and stress were the major causes of heart disease [27]. In a sample of patients who had experienced an AMI, diet and smoking were most frequently stated as causes of heart disease [30]. Women who experienced an AMI were more aware of the causes of CAD than men [27].

Both men and women were unable to correctly identify the leading causes of an AMI.

Discussion

The purpose of this report was to synthesize and critically analyze gender differences in knowledge, attitudes, and beliefs about heart disease. Studies of women only and studies of both men and women were included in this research. Comparison of knowledge, attitudes, and beliefs about heart disease both supported and refuted current perceptions.

Lack of consistent conceptual or operational definitions of knowledge, attitudes, or beliefs about heart disease was striking. Researchers were not consistent in listing traditional risk factors for CAD, typical and atypical symptoms of AMI, or questions concerning attitudes and beliefs about CAD. The lack of consistent definitions for all the constructs investigated made it difficult to compare the results of these studies and limited the generalizability of the findings. This can also add to public's confusion in identifying significant risk factors, signs, and symptoms of AMI, and appropriate interventions for reducing risks for CAD.

Differences in research designs added to the difficulty in comparing results across studies. This review included 14 studies of women only and 24 studies of both men and women. In the studies of only women, the majority (50%) were surveys conducted through random-digit dialing. In 21% of the studies, data were collected through mail surveys, and 29% of surveys were conducted through in-person interviews. In contrast, the majority (75%) of studies of both men and women were face-to-face interviews; only 13% of the studies used random-digit dialing surveys, and there was one mailed survey.

Each study design has inherent problems. Information obtained in a mailed survey may differ from information obtained in face-to-face interviews. A likelihood in face-to-face interviews is that the respondent provides an answer they think the researcher wants to hear instead of what they really believe. Differences in the sampling design can also lead to problems. Selection bias may be present in telephone surveys because persons of lower socioeconomic status, or ethnic minorities may not have telephone service and therefore are not able to participate.

In the studies of women only, 71% (10) were surveys of the general public, 21% (3) of the studies were of women with CAD, and 7% (1) study was of women with a history of breast cancer. In contrast, 58% (14) of the studies of both men and women were surveys of the general public, 33% (8) of studies were conducted among men and women with known CAD, and 4% (1) survey was of smokers. Knowledge level may be different in each group based on personal experiences.

These differences in methodology limit the generalizability of these findings. There was no consistent focus on one aspect of heart disease, and often questionnaires included many other topics than knowledge, attitudes, and beliefs about heart disease. Therefore, only parts of the study were included in the comparison of the results. There was no consistent questionnaire or set of questions used to measure knowledge, attitudes, or beliefs, which also limited the ability to compare the results.

Despite a number of limitations in this body of literature, certain conclusions can be drawn. The identification of heart disease as the leading cause of death in men and women has improved over time but still is suboptimal in both men and women [2,3,12,13]. Although chest pain was the most commonly recognized symptom of an AMI by both men and women

[18,20,22], atypical symptoms were not well recognized, and people were unsure of how they should respond to symptoms of an AMI, often delaying seeking care [5]. This latter finding is of concern because accumulating evidence suggests that most people of either gender do not have severe "typical" chest pain and often experience atypical symptoms. If people are not able to recognize the signs and symptoms of an AMI, appropriate action cannot be taken in a timely manner, negatively affecting treatment options.

The majority of women did not know that heart disease is the leading cause of death in women [3,6,10]. Although there has been an increase in awareness since the early 1990s, women still consider heart disease to be a man's disease, even when they have a strong family history of CAD [4,22,29]. Women also tend to believe they are not at risk for an AMI [4,35]. Older women often worried less about heart disease than younger women did [33]. Breast cancer is still the health risk that worries most women [2,3].

Both men and women had poor spontaneous recall of risk factors for CAD and AMI. Women were better able to recognize risk factors if they were given a list [7]. Men and women often underestimated their risk for CAD, and high-risk individuals with known heart disease also underestimated their future risk for CAD [4,6,29,35]. Women's belief about their risk for CAD was addressed in 3 studies of women with known heart disease [4,26,44]. All reported that only a minority of high-risk women believed they were at risk for CAD. King and colleagues [34] reported that 84% of women studied reported 3 or more individual risk factors, but only 33% of the women stated they had been told they were at risk for CAD. Age influenced whether women remembered being told they were at risk for CAD; 53% of women less than age 44 recalled being told they were at risk compared with 32% of women aged 60 and older. Having a personal history of CAD did not influence whether women remembered being told they were at risk for CAD. People with known CAD who had undergone treatment, believed they were no longer at risk for future events and often delayed until they had severe symptoms before seeking care [5]. If individuals do not believe they are at risk for CAD/AMI, they are less likely to adopt a healthy lifestyle.

College-age men and women both underestimated their risk and were incorrect in their assumptions about the leading cause of death in women [14,28]. Understanding risks for CAD at an earlier age may lead to better health knowledge and lifestyle modifications to alter health risks. The paucity of studies comparing gender and age as well as studies in young people precluded comparisons of men and women, specific ethnic groups, or younger versus older individuals.

Men and women often did not have a plan for what they would do in the event of an AMI [22]. The majority of men and women were with others when symptoms of AMI occurred and discussed their symptoms before seeking care for those symptoms [22]. Most men and women who sought medical care for symptoms of an AMI did not attribute the symptoms they were experiencing to the heart [22,29]. Many individuals delayed seeking care until their symptoms worsened. African-American and Hispanic women delayed longer than other groups [22]. Women who had undergone CABG or PCI delayed seeking care for symptoms of AMI because they no longer perceived themselves to be a risk for CAD; they did not seek care until symptoms became unbearable [5].

More than 90% of individuals say they would act quickly in response to symptoms of an AMI and call 911 [15,16,18]. Almost all women (93%) reported if they or someone they knew experienced symptoms of a heart attack, the most important thing to do was get to the hospital [16]. A total of 86% of women said the most important thing to do was to call 911 [16]. However, what individuals say they would do contradicts the fact that most individuals delay seeking care for their symptoms [22,29]. Only 11% of Greenlund and colleagues' sample and 20% of Meischke and colleagues' sample called 911 if someone were having symptoms of a heart attack [17,18]. Often women wanted to be sure they were having a heart attack before going to the emergency room, and more women chose to go to the emergency room by their own means rather than call 911 [15]. Delay in seeking care for symptoms of AMI impacts morbidity and mortality.

Practice implications

Understanding the current lack of knowledge and attitudes and beliefs about heart disease by both men and women will provide health care providers with an opportunity to address individual as well as community health risks. Several studies reported that very few people recalled being told they were at risk for CAD despite family histories and personal risk factors for CAD. However, knowledge alone is not sufficient to change behavior. Understanding a person's beliefs and attitudes about their risk for CAD will allow the provider to tailor the information given to patients to better persuade individuals to adopt healthy lifestyles and appropriate responses to signs and symptoms of CAD.

National campaigns by the American Heart Association (AHA), including the Red Dress symbol for women and heart disease, are attempting to raise public awareness about heart disease for both men and women. Written information as well as discussions about CAD prevention strategies, risk stratification, risk factors, signs and symptoms of AMI, and, as appropriate, responses to symptoms should be part of primary health care delivery. Information about heart disease should be addressed at annual examinations and on regular visits with individuals at risk for development of CAD.

Education of health care providers is also critical in the fight to reduce morbidity and mortality from CAD. Formal as well as informal education is needed to raise awareness of prevention strategies, risk factor identification, and treatment options. The treatment and management of CAD is an ever-changing field, and practitioners need to remain current to better care for their patients. The development of effective counseling strategies is a key in decreasing morbidity and mortality from CAD.

Research implications

Researchers need to come to consensus on the best definitions of the concepts of knowledge, attitudes, and beliefs about heart disease and methodologies to better understand their interrelationships. Agreement of key variables would allow comparisons of research findings. Not all investigators described age, gender, education, socioeconomic status, or ethnic/racial differences. The inclusion of these variables in the questionnaires would allow researchers to determine similarities as well as differences between the groups. Sample selection that addresses these characteristics will allow a better identification and understanding of at-risk groups. Understanding the similarities and differences would provide opportunities to develop targeted interventions at high-risk groups.

Many of the investigators developed their own questionnaires that were a combination of open-ended questions, Likert-type scales, or lists of symptoms to elicit the information, and the data were collected in a variety of ways. Questions ranged from concerns about heart disease, to perceptions of personal or general risk for CAD, to the probability of developing CAD, to causes of heart disease. There was no consistency in the list of risk factors, typical and atypical symptoms of coronary heart disease (CHD), or questions about attitudes or beliefs about heart disease.

The use of Likert-type scales, list of items, or closed-ended questions in a questionnaire forces the participant to choose from the items listed and is more likely to measure recognition, whereas open-ended questions measure recall. The ability to recall facts may indicate understanding of the concept being measured. Depending on the concept to be measured, each type of question has advantages and disadvantages. For example, if measuring knowledge of heart disease as the leading cause of death with a yes or no response, the participant has to make a choice recalling what he or she knows or remembers. If the participant is asked what they believe is the leading cause of death, he or she can respond with a belief, and it may or may not assess knowledge.

Consensus regarding lists of risk factors for CAD and signs and symptoms of AMI, would allow comparison of results and identification of areas of deficit. The AHA has identified a list of risk factors for CAD based on research findings. If researchers consistently used those risk factors in their research, making comparisons of the findings would be more meaningful.

Mail surveys, telephone interviews, and face-to-face interviews were conducted with structured and semistructured questions to obtain the information. There is no ideal method to obtain the answers to the questions of interest. Understanding the benefits and limitations of each method should drive the decision regarding which survey method to use.

A limitation of all studies is the accuracy and reliability of the answers to the questions. Few investigators described instrument development or psychometric properties of the instruments used to collect the data. The development and reporting of the psychometric properties of an instrument may encourage other researchers to use valid and reliable tools in their assessment of knowledge, attitudes, and beliefs. Repeated use of a questionnaire allows comparisons of data. Identifying deficits in knowledge, attitudes, and beliefs about heart disease will provide opportunities to develop targeted interventions for high-risk groups.

Summary

The purpose of this study was to synthesize and critically analyze knowledge, attitudes, and beliefs about heart disease. Both men and women had low levels of knowledge of symptoms and risk factors of heart disease, and they underestimated their risk for cardiac events. Women's knowledge about heart disease was not worse than men's. Women showed more knowledge concerning less common symptoms of AMI. Heart disease was seen as a man's disease, and women were more concerned about breast cancer than heart disease. Men and women recognized the need to seek immediate care for symptoms of AMI, but research to date does not show that they indeed take such action; individuals delay, on average, more than 2 hours before seeking care [31]. There are insufficient data to identify the influence of gender, age, and ethnicity on knowledge, attitudes, and beliefs about heart disease. The magnitude of this problem necessitates the need for focused efforts to address these deficits.

References

[1] American Heart Association. Heart Disease and Stroke Statistics - 2006 Update 2006.

[2] Mosca L, Jones WK, King KB, et al. Awareness, perception, and knowledge of heart disease risk and prevention among women in the United States. Arch Fam Med 2000;9(6): 506–15.

[3] Mosca L, Ferris A, Fabunmi R, et al. Tracking women's awareness of heart disease: an American Heart Association national study. Circulation 2004;109(5):573–9.

[4] Marcuccio E, Loving N, Bennett SK, et al. A survey of attitudes and experiences of women with heart disease. Womens Health Issues 2003;13(1):23–31.

[5] Pattenden J, Watt I, Lewin RJ, et al. Decision making processes in people with symptoms of acute myocardial infarction: qualitative study. BMJ 2002;324(7344):1006–9.

[6] Wilcox S, Stefanick ML. Knowledge and perceived risk of major diseases in middle-aged and older women. Health Psychol 1999;18(4):346–53.

[7] Andersson P, Leppert J. Men of low socio-economic and educational level possess pronounced deficient knowledge about the risk factors related to coronary heart disease. J Cardiovasc Risk 2001;8(6):371–7.

[8] Cambridge Dictionary. 2005.
[9] Green LW, Kreuter MW. Health Program Planning: An Educational and Ecological Approach. 4th edition. New York: McGraw-Hill; 2005.
[10] Prendergast HM, Bunney EB, Roberson T, et al. Knowledge of heart disease among women in an urban emergency setting. J Natl Med Assoc 2004;96(8):1027–31.
[11] Meischke H, Sellers DE, Robbins ML, et al. Factors that influence personal perceptions of the risk of an acute myocardial infarction. Behav Med 2000;26(1):4–13.
[12] Erhardt L, Hobbs FD. Public perceptions of cardiovascular risk in five European countries: the react survey. Int J Clin Pract 2002;56(9):638–44.
[13] Shepherd J, Alcalde V, Befort PA, et al. International comparison of awareness and attitudes towards coronary risk factor reduction: the HELP study. J Cardiovasc Risk 1997;4(5/6): 373–84.
[14] Collins KM, Dantico M, Shearer NBC, et al. Heart disease awareness among college students. J Community Health 2004;29(5):405–20.
[15] Wyatt P, Ratner P. Evaluating treatment-seeking for acute myocardial infarction in women. Can J Cardiovasc Nurs 2004;14(1):39–45.
[16] Meischke H, Kuniyuki MS, Yasui Y, et al. Information women receive about heart attacks and how it affects their knowledge, beliefs, and intentions to act in a cardiac emergency. Health Care Women Int 2002;23:149–62.
[17] Meischke H, Yasui Y, Kuniyuki A, et al. How women label and respond to symptoms of acute myocardial infarction: responses to hypothetical symptom scenarios. Heart Lung 1999;28(4):261–9.
[18] Greenlund KJ, Keenan NL, Giles WH, et al. Public recognition of major signs and symptoms of heart attack: seventeen states and the US Virgin Islands, 2001. Am Heart J 2004; 147(6):1010–6.
[19] Zerwic JJ. Symptoms of acute myocardial infarction: expectations of a community sample. Heart Lung 1998;27(2):75–81.
[20] Goff DC Jr, Sellers DE, McGovern PG, et al. Knowledge of heart attack symptoms in a population survey in the United States: The REACT Trial. Rapid Early Action for Coronary Treatment. Arch Intern Med 1998;158(21):2329–38.
[21] Johnson JA, King KB. Influence of expectations about symptoms on delay in seeking treatment during myocardial infarction. Am J Crit Care 1995;4(1):29–35.
[22] Finnegan JR Jr, Meischke H, Zapka JG, et al. Patient delay in seeking care for heart attack symptoms: findings from focus groups conducted in five U.S. regions. Prev Med 2000;31(3): 205–13.
[23] Tullmann D, Dracup K. Knowledge of heart attack symptoms in older man and women at risk for acute myocardial infarction. J Cardpulm Rehabil 2005;25:33–9.
[24] Goff DC Jr, Feldman HA, McGovern PG, et al. Prehospital delay in patients hospitalized with heart attack symptoms in the United States: the REACT trial. Rapid Early Action for Coronary Treatment (REACT) Study Group. Am Heart J 1999;138(6 Pt 1):1046–57.
[25] Momtahan K, Berkman J, Sellick J, et al. Patients' understanding of cardiac risk factors: a point-prevalence study. J Cardiovasc Nurs 2004;19(1):13–20.
[26] Oliver-McNeil SA, Artinian NT. Women's perception of personal cardiovascular risk and their risk-reducing behaviors. Am J Crit Care 2002;11(3):221–7.
[27] Kirkland SA, MacLean DR, Langille DB, et al. Knowledge and awareness of risk factors for cardiovascular disease among Canadians 55 to 74 years of age: results from the Canadian Heart Health Surveys, 1986–1992. Can Med Assoc J 1999;161(Suppl 8):S10–6.
[28] Green JS, Grant M, Hill KL, et al. Heart disease risk perception in college men and women. J Am Coll Health 2003;51(5):207–11.
[29] Van Tiel D, van Vliet KP, Moerman CJ. Sex differences in illness beliefs and illness behavior in patients with suspected coronary artery disease. Patient Educ Couns 1998;33(2):143–7.
[30] Zerwic JJ, King KB, Wlasowicz GS. Perceptions of patients with cardiovascular disease about the causes of coronary artery disease. Heart Lung 1997;26(2):92–8.

[31] Moser DK, McKinley S, Dracup K, et al. Gender differences in reasons patients delay in seeking treatment for acute myocardial infarction symptoms. Patient Educ Couns 2005; 56(1):45–54.

[32] King R. Illness attributions and myocardial infarction: the influence of gender and socio-economic circumstances on illness beliefs. J Adv Nurs 2002;37(5):431–8.

[33] Biswas MS, Calhoun PS, Bosworth HB, et al. Are women worrying about heart disease? Women's Health Issues 2002;12(4):204–11.

[34] King KB, Quinn JR, Delehanty JM, et al. Perception of risk for coronary heart disease in women undergoing coronary angiography. Heart Lung 2002;31(4):246–52.

[35] Legato MJ, Padus E, Slaughter E. Women's perceptions of their general health, with special reference to their risk of coronary artery disease: results of a national telephone survey. J Womens Health 1997;6(2):189–98.

[36] Meischke H, Eisenberg M, Schaeffer S, et al. The 'Heart Attack Survival Kit' project: an intervention designed to increase seniors' intentions to respond appropriately to symptoms of acute myocardial infarction. Health Educ Res 2000;15(3):317–26.

[37] Frijling BD, Lobo CM, Keus IM, et al. Perceptions of cardiovascular risk among patients with hypertension or diabetes. Patient Educ Couns 2004;52(1):47–53.

[38] Ayanian J, Cleary P. Perceived risks of heart disease and cancer among cigarette smokers. JAMA 1999;281(11):1019–21.

[39] Ferrario G, Alkhimovitch O, Avanzini F, et al. People's perception of their overall coronary risk: an Italian experience. Ital Heart J 2004;5(1):16–21.

[40] McDermott MM, Mandapat AL, Moates A, et al. Knowledge and attitudes regarding cardiovascular disease risk and prevention in patients with coronary or peripheral arterial disease. Arch Intern Med 2003;163(18):2157–62.

[41] Montgomery GH, Erblich J, DiLorenzo T, et al. Family and friends with disease: their impact on perceived risk. Prev Med 2003;37(3):242–9.

[42] Erblich J, Bovbjerg DH, Norman C, et al. It won't happen to me: lower perception of heart disease risk among women with family histories of breast cancer. Prev Med 2000;31(6): 714–21.

[43] Murray S. The interplay between social and cultural context and perceptions of cardiovascular disease. J Adv Nurs 2000;32(5):1224–33.

[44] King KM, Arthur HM. Coronary heart disease prevention: views on women's gender-based perceptions and meanings. J Cardiovasc Nurs 2003;18(4):274–81.

[45] Pilote L, Hlatky M. Attitudes of women toward hormone therapy and prevention of heart disease. American Heart Journal 1995;129(6):1237–8.

NURSING
CLINICS
OF NORTH AMERICA

Nurs Clin N Am 43 (2008) 105–115

The Effects of a Mediterranean-Style Dietary Pattern on Cardiovascular Disease Risk

Frances Hardin-Fanning, RN, MSN

College of Nursing, University of Kentucky, 760 Rose Street, HSLC 450B, Lexington, KY 40356, USA

A third of all American adults have at least one type of cardiovascular disease (CVD), and the lifetime risk for CVD is two in three for men and greater than one in two for women at age 40. On average, CVD causes one death every 36 seconds in the United States [1]. Risk factor modification is crucial to decreasing cardiovascular morbidity and mortality. Nine risk factors account for 90% of CVD risk: (1) smoking, (2) hypertension, (3) type 2 diabetes mellitus, (4) waist-to-hip ratio, (5) dietary patterns, (6) physical activity, (7) alcohol consumption, (8) ratio of apolipoprotein (apo) B to apo A-1, and (9) psychosocial factors). Eight of these factors are influenced by nutritional habits [2].

The typical Western diet is high in refined starches, sugar, and saturated fats that actively increase the risk of cardiovascular disease [3]. It can be difficult for individuals to identify the most effective nutritional alternatives to the Western diet. Consumers are faced with choosing from a myriad of nutraceuticals, supplements, and diet programs, often with conflicting reports as to the benefits and risks. Medications and supplements that are marketed for CVD risk reduction have been discovered later to have minimal or even unfavorable health effects. Individuals of lower socioeconomic status, who have the highest degree of CVD risk, are also the least able to afford supplements and fortified food products marketed as heart-healthy [4].

Mediterranean-style diets (MD) contain many of the nutrients known to decrease CVD. These include foods with limited saturated and trans fats and adequate omega-3 polyunsaturated fatty acids (PUFA), such as fruits, vegetables, nuts, and whole grains [3,5]. The MD meets the current dietary recommendations for CVD risk reduction in healthy, at-risk, and

E-mail address: fdbowe2@email.uky.edu

chronically ill adults [6–9]. The diet also meets recommendations for fiber (20 to 30 g) and cholesterol (<200 mg) intake [10]. Following an MD can result in significant decreases in body weight, body mass index (BMI), waist circumference, blood pressure, glucose, insulin, total cholesterol, triglycerides, and proinflammatory cytokines, and can increase high-density lipoprotein (HDL) cholesterol in people who have metabolic syndrome [7]. Further, the diet has shown no adverse effects in any population, and is cost-effective, with high rates of adherence, making it an ideal alternative to the typical Western diet. Therefore, this article describes the role of key nutrients in the MD in the prevention of atherogenesis in moderate- to high-risk populations.

Mediterranean-style diet

The Mediterranean-style diet is not a specific diet, but rather a collection of eating habits traditionally followed by people in the 16 countries surrounding the Mediterranean Sea. Although specific nutrients in the diet have shown a propensity for decreasing cardiovascular risk, the most significant effects have been noted when key nutrients are a part of a dietary pattern. It is the synergistic, antagonistic, and complementary effects of these nutrients that contribute to the inhibitory effects of the diet on atherogenesis [2,5,6,8–10]. Individuals who adhere to an MD have lower proinflammatory markers, which are indicative of lower CVD risk, than those who simply supplement their usual diet with foods (ie, beans, tomatoes, whole grains) that are known to have anti-atherogenic properties [6]. Although it appears the combination of nutrients in the MD is most important, an understanding of the roles that specific nutrients play in the development and prevention of CVD is essential in guiding food choice for anyone considering adopting the MD.

Role of dietary fats in cardiovascular pathophysiology

Lipids

Lipids, particularly cholesterol, contribute to vascular endothelial dysfunction. Low-density lipoprotein (LDL), the major carrier of cholesterol, is transported to the liver and peripheral tissues via the transport protein apo B-100. LDL and apo B-100 bind with receptors located on the endothelial cell surface, and the entire particle is internalized by the cells. Once inside the cell, the receptor releases LDL and returns to the cell surface to bind and transport additional LDL. Within the cell, LDL is processed into amino acids, free fatty acids, and free cholesterol to perform normal physiological functions. When levels of LDL are high, however, they initiate oxidation, inflammation, and development of foam cells, which are lipid-engorged phagocytic cells, all of which increase the risk for CVD [11].

In contrast, HDL reduce CVD risk is several ways. First, HDL binds with both the HDL specific receptor, apo E, and to the LDL receptor, apo B-100. Therefore, HDL competes with LDL for the apo B-100 receptor, resulting in less LDL entering the cell. Second, HDL transports LDL to the liver for reprocessing and excretion. Third, HDL stimulates the enzyme lecithin, which transforms free cholesterol into cholesteryl esters that are more readily transported to the liver an excreted as bile salt. The net result is less LDL-mediated endothelial damage and subsequent development of atherosclerosis.

The amount of specific dietary fatty acids in the diet influences the proportion of LDL to HDL cholesterol. Diets with higher amounts of PUFA and monounsaturated fatty acids (MUFA) result in LDL/HDL ratios that are protective against CVD, whereas saturated fatty acids produce ratios that promote CVD [11]. In addition to increasing HDL levels, PUFA have other cardioprotective effects.

Polyunsaturated Fatty Acids

Omega-3 and omega-6 PUFA are considered essential because humans are unable to synthesize these fatty acids, and therefore are required to obtain them through the diet. The three most important dietary omega-3 PUFA are α-linolenic acid (ALA), which is derived mainly from seed oils, and eicosapentaenoic acid (EPA) and docosahexaenoic acid (DHA), which are found mainly in fatty fish, including wild salmon, herring, mackerel, anchovies, tuna, and sardines. Plant-sources of omega-3 fatty acids include walnuts, tofu, and some leafy green vegetables. Sources of omega-6 fatty acids include corn, safflower, sunflower, and soybean oils. A ratio of omega-6 to omega-3 of 4:1 is associated with nearly a 70% decrease in total CVD mortality [12]. Unfortunately, current Western dietary patterns contain ratios of omega-6 to omega-3 fatty acids as high as 17:1 [13]. This ratio tips metabolic pathways in favor of omega-6 PUFA. Omega-6 PUFA compete with omega-3 PUFA for integration into all body cell membranes. These two fatty acids are metabolically distinct with opposing physiological functions. Although both omega-6 and omega-3 PUFA can have some positive effects on lipids, omega-6 fatty acids negatively impact vascular endothelium by promoting production of eicosanoid inflammatory mediators. Eicosanoids are metabolites of PUFA that are synthesized by the cyclooxygenase, epoxygenases, and lipoxygenase pathways. These metabolites are formed into prostaglandins, thromboxanes, lipoxins, and leukotrienes, all of which are involved in the inflammatory processes. Eicosanoid production is stimulated either physiologically or pathologically, such as in ischemia or mechanical damage. The metabolism of omega-6 PUFA forms larger amounts of proinflammatory and prothrombotic metabolites [11,14,15]. In contrast, omega-3 PUFA produce metabolites with vascular endothelial protective properties that reduce the risk of inflammatory-mediated cardiovascular disease [11,14,15]. Diets high in omega-3 PUFA also reduce cardiovascular mortality by lowering blood pressure and cholesterol, inhibiting platelet aggregation, and exerting antiarrhythmic effects. They also improve lipid profiles and endothelial function [16].

Higher levels of omega-3 PUFA are also associated with secondary prevention. Postmenopausal women who have coronary artery disease and who had DHA above median in their cohort had significantly less progression of coronary atherosclerosis and fewer new lesions over 3 years than those who had lower levels [17]. In a 6-week, randomized, controlled crossover study of male patients who had heart failure, dietary omega-3 fatty acids (fish oil) supplementation enhanced endothelium-dependent vasodilation and decreased serum triglyceride levels [18]. This enhanced endothelium-dependent vasodilation is particularly important in CVD risk, because impaired endothelium vasodilation is associated with a relative risk of 4.65 for cardiovascular events [19]. In a case-control analysis, individuals who had confirmed myocardial infarction, unstable angina pectoris, or acute coronary syndrome had significantly lower levels of EPA/DHA in cell membranes than individuals who did not have CVD. Lower blood EPA/DHA content was an independent predictor of increased risk of cardiovascular events in the individuals who had CVD [20]. Interestingly, there were no differences in trans fatty acids levels between the cases and controls. Further, higher blood trans fatty acid level did not predict CVD. This observation is of interest given the recent attention to the association of trans fatty acids with CVD risk.

It is important to note that a limitation of most studies involving omega-3 supplementation was the lack of dietary pattern analysis. The data suggest that changes in the whole diet toward eating patterns consistent with the MD yield significantly more improvement in CVD outcomes and prevention [8]. This pattern should include fatty fish if possible. Evidence is mounting that marine-source DHA may be the most important omega-3 fatty acid for reducing CVD risk. The data suggest that fish oils result in higher levels of DHA in cell membranes than flaxseed oil [21]. For example, the amount of EPA and DHA contained in 6 oz or more of fatty fish per week can reduce the risk of cardiac death by 36% and total mortality by 17%. The American Heart Association (AHA) recommends 1 g of dietary omega-3 fatty acids per day for secondary prevention of cardiac disease. This amount is equivalent to 4 servings of omega-3–rich fish per week. Intake of 250 to 500 mg per day of EPA and DHA is sufficient for primary prevention, whereas 2 to 3 g of ALA per day are required to obtain a similar level of prevention [22].

Omega-9 Monounsaturated Fatty Acids

Other fats in the MD potentiate the cardio-protective effects of omega-3 PUFA. In particular, the omega-9 MUFA oleic acid, which is a major component of olive oil, is recognized to have complementary cardio-protective benefits. Omega-9 MUFA inhibit the inflammatory process that results from LDL oxidation and endothelial activation. Animal and human studies have demonstrated that olive oil improves cardiovascular function by significantly decreasing atherosclerosis, hypertension, hypercholesterolemia, and diabetes [23].

Antioxidant polyphenols

Olive oil, fruits, and vegetables are consumed in moderate to large quantities in the MD. The phenols, or chemical substances found in these foods, have synergistic effects when combined with omega-3 fatty acids. Epidemiologic studies show an inverse relationship between dietary intake of polyphenols and CVD risk [24]. Polyphenols are found in all plant species, but are found in high amounts in olive oil. The majority of dietary polyphenols are in the form of flavonoids, which decrease the risk of CVD through several mechanisms. Polyphenols appear to reduce absorption of cholesterol by interacting with transport molecules across the brush border of the gastrointestinal (GI) tract. This reduced absorption of cholesterol generates a dose-response up-regulation of LDL receptors, resulting in lower plasma cholesterol levels. Polyphenols also affect hepatic production of lipoproteins and decrease plasma triglyceride and apo B concentrations. Other possible actions of polyphenols include the scavenging of free radicals produced during normal physiological functions, removal of pro-oxidant ions, recycling of vitamin E α-tocopherol, preservation of HDL activity, inhibition of cellular enzymes responsible for LDL oxidation, and inhibition of proinflammatory pathways [25]. The overall effects of dietary polyphenols are reduced plasma LDL cholesterol and triglycerides, and improved endothelial function. Polyphenols also inhibit inflammation by decreasing monocyte and T-lymphocyte adhesion molecules, tumor necrosis factor-alpha (TNFα), interleukin (IL)-6, and arterial wall cellular adhesion molecules [26].

Several wild greens that are indigenous to the Mediterranean area are very high in phenolic compounds and exert powerful antioxidant properties. Although there are several antioxidant-rich fruits and vegetables grown in the United States, the majority of dietary polyphenol flavonoids in the American diet come from tea, wine, and citrus fruits and juices [27]. Nearly 78% of American adults consume less than five servings of fruits and vegetables daily [1]. Vegetable sources of flavonoids in the United States include spinach, collard, kale, Brussels sprouts, broccoli, alfalfa sprouts, bell peppers, and onions. Fruits sources include prunes, raisins, blueberries, blackberries, strawberries, and raspberries.

Vitamin antioxidants

Vitamin E includes eight compounds, with α-tocopherol being the most biologically active form. Synthetic forms of the vitamin, found in supplements and fortified foods, are not as active and have an established tolerable upper limit of 1 g daily for adults. Vitamin E protects the cell membrane by preventing lipid oxidation through inhibition of free radical and singlet molecular oxygen reactions. Free radicals, which are atoms or molecules with unpaired electrons, are produced during many body processes and are highly reactive. Free radicals damage the lipid component cell membranes by taking electrons from PUFA membrane. This process has been implicated in many chronic diseases, including CVD [28,29]. Plasma LDL particles are protected from oxidation by antioxidants, including α-tocopherol, through the scavenging of free radicals. During unsaturation of PUFA, vitamin E requirements increase. Fortunately, foods high in PUFA and MUFA also are good sources of vitamin E, and absorption of vitamin E is more efficient when consumed with dietary fats.

α-tocopherol, found in many plant oils, including olive oil, is the most abundant antioxidant in the diet. Under certain circumstances, α-tocopherol can also act as a pro-oxidant; however, ascorbic acid, found in fruits and vegetables, can inhibit this pro-oxidant activity by regenerating the α-tocopherol molecule. Yet, in some studies, supplemental ascorbic acid also reacted as a pro-oxidant in the late phases of lipid oxidation [28].

Epidemiologic studies show that foods rich in antioxidants are associated with reduced CVD, but intervention trials using supplements have not yielded similar results. In contrast, interventional trials with whole food sources of antioxidants show reductions in plasma concentrations of inflammatory biomarkers and oxidized LDL, improvement in lipoprotein profile, and favor a reduction in CVD risk [30]. Foods rich in antioxidants also have high levels of polyphenols, and this may be the reason for decreased CVD risk in individuals who adhere to an MD.

Current evidence is insufficient to support recommendations either for or against the use of multivitamin/mineral supplements for primary or secondary prevention of cardiovascular disease [31]. Nutrient intake from food is incremental over several meals and is not comparable to supplemental intake in a single dose. Food sources of antioxidants and vitamins, with the exception of folic acid, generally have greater bioavailability than supplemental sources. Combined, these observations further emphasize the importance of making whole dietary pattern changes rather than simply focusing on supplementing one or several dietary nutrients to improve outcomes.

Folic acid

Food sources of folic acid include green vegetables, mushrooms, legumes, peanuts, and fruits. Raw foods are typically higher in folic acid than cooked foods, because up to 95% of natural folic acid can be lost during cooking. Folic acid functions as a coenzyme in many physiological processes and, along with vitamins B_6 and B_{12}, is instrumental in the amino acid conversion of homocysteine to methionine. Hyperhomocysteinemia, a pro-oxidative, proinflammatory, and prothrombotic condition, contributes to endothelial dysfunction, and is associated with increased CVD risk in middle-aged and older adults. High levels of homocysteine pose as great a risk factor for CVD as elevated LDL cholesterol. Studies of synthetic folic acid supplementation to reduce hyperhomocysteinemia have had mixed results. Although folic acid is necessary for homocysteine conversion, current evidence does not support recommendations for supplements or fortified foods to decrease CVD risk [1,30]. In some studies, synthetic folic acid actually increased the risk of CVD when given in combination with other vitamins [32].

Folic acid has other health-related effects that merit discussion in relationship to the MD. Atrophic gastritis, the cause of B_{12} anemia, affects up to 50% of older adults and predisposes them to gastric cancer. Atrophic gastritis is influenced by proinflammatory cytokines and prostaglandins, and levels of these molecules are lower in individuals whose diets are more similar to an MD [6,9]. This inflammatory process is characterized by a partial loss of fundic glands and decrease in parietal cell mass, resulting in a loss of the intrinsic factor necessary for B_{12} absorption.

Folic acid supplementation can mask megaloblastic macrocytic anemia of vitamin B_{12} deficiency, allowing neurological damage to occur. Because it can be several years before the B_{12} deficiency anemia manifests, older adults who take synthetic folic acid are at higher risk for irreversible neurological impairment caused by a B_{12} deficiency. For this reason, a tolerable upper intake level of 1 mg synthetic folic acid from supplements or fortified foods is recommended [33].

Folic acid in foods exists in polyglutamate forms, and must be metabolized by the body to a monoglutamate form. During this conversion, a significant amount of folic acid is lost. Synthetic folic acid, found in supplements and fortified foods, is already in the monoglutamate form and does not undergo this process. The greater bioavailability of supplemental folic acid increases blood levels and subsequently the risk for masked vitamin B_{12} anemia [33]. Because of very low bioavailability, there is no tolerable upper limit for natural folic acid derived from food. Adherence to an MD is associated with incrementally lower serum levels of homocysteine, indicating that supplementation is not necessary with a proper diet. Thus, the folic acid present in an MD may be a much more appropriate source for CVD risk reduction than supplemental folic acid.

Fiber

Fiber, which is a plant carbohydrate material, is abundant in the MD in the form of grains, fruits, and vegetables. Humans digest carbohydrates through the enzymatic activity of salivary α-amylase on the carbohydrate molecule's α-glycosidic bonds. Plant fiber has β-glycosidic bonds that are resistant to α-amylase, and passes through the GI tract intact. These fiber molecules are able to bind with cholesterol and prevent absorption in the small intestine. In the colon, the bound cholesterol is either excreted in feces or is degraded by intestinal bacteria. This process results in a decreased amount of LDL cholesterol undergoing enterohepatic recirculation, which promotes removal of LDL cholesterol from the blood for bile synthesis, thereby reducing serum LDL cholesterol and decreasing CVD risk [34].

Americans consume an average of 15 g of the recommended 25 g of fiber daily, and most consume less than 1 serving of whole grains each day [1]. High dietary fiber is also associated with decreased inflammatory markers. Diets that contain high fiber foods such as fruit, nuts, and cereal, are associated with lower concentrations of IL-6, indicating lower levels of inflammatory activity in the body [35]. Whole grain foods also contain antioxidants, folic acid, and phenolic compounds, which contribute to a reduced risk of CVD. Nuts and seeds, which are high in fiber, PUFA, MUFA, vitamins, and antioxidants, improve plasma lipid profiles and endothelial function, and inhibit platelet aggregation and inflammation.

Alcohol

Another component of the MD is alcohol in moderation. Mechanisms for protective effect of alcohol on the cardiovascular system include elevation of HDL, lower serum low-density cholesterol, and the inhibition of endothelial smooth muscle cell proliferation that occurs during atherogenesis. Individuals who consume moderate amounts of alcohol have lower levels of acute phase proteins and proinflammatory cytokines than non-drinkers or heavy drinkers. Moderate alcohol intake also inhibits insulin resistance by regulating enzyme activity during glycolysis and increasing antioxidant capacity to protect cells against oxidative stress. Reservatrol, found in red wine, inhibits lipogenesis and platelet aggregation. Red wine also contains powerful antioxidant polyphenols that exhibit endothelium-dependent vasodilatation properties and attenuation of cells involved in the proinflammatory response [36]. Thus, moderate alcohol intake results in cardiovascular benefits because of a healthier vascular endothelium, and these results are greater when associated with an MD [37].

High doses of alcohol initiate the acute phase response after an initial suppression, whereas low doses actually inhibit acute phase responses induced by other stimuli [38]. For this reason, alcohol should be consumed in small to moderate amounts daily, and not ingested in larger quantities on an occasional basis. Alcohol is quickly absorbed in the GI tract and oxidized by alcohol dehydrogenase (ADH), which is present in the gastric mucosal cells and the cytoplasm of the liver cells. There is a significant gender difference in the activity of ADH in the gastric mucosal cells, with women having much less ADH activity. Therefore, women develop higher blood alcohol levels and are a greater risk of hepatotoxicity than men who drink the same amount of alcohol. Consequently, women should consume one drink per day, and men two drinks per day to achieve the cardiovascular benefits of ethanol. A drink is defined as 12 oz. of beer, 4 oz of wine, or 1 to 1.5 oz of liquor [39].

Summary

Evidence supports reduced CVD incidence with adherence to an MD. Omega-3 PUFA and MUFA, antioxidants, fiber, folic acid, and alcohol are some of the important components of this dietary pattern. Each of these nutrients plays a key role in the inhibition of atherogenesis and the protection of vascular endothelial cells. When nutrients are combined in the diet, they exhibit synergistic and antagonistic properties. Different foods in the diet are able to impact CVD risk at various points in the atherogenic process, and the whole-diet approach to prevention is synergistic for maximum effect. Supplementing single nutrients in otherwise unhealthy dietary pattern does not provide the same cardiovascular protection, and in certain circumstances can be harmful. From clinical observations, supplements often are perceived as implicit permission to maintain or resume unhealthy eating patterns.

Adherence to an MD results in lower circulating LDL cholesterol and triglycerides, elevated HDL cholesterol, impedance of LDL oxidation, protection of the endothelium, inhibition of inflammatory and eicosanoid molecules responsible for cell damage, improved glucose use, and lower blood pressure. The MD is cost-effective for primary and secondary prevention, has moderate adherence rates, and its components are readily available to most Americans because of global trade. Populations most at risk for CVD also tend to be of lower socioeconomic status, and often have limited resources for primary disease prevention. Despite these barriers, effective nutritional counseling can produce changes in dietary patterns that decrease CVD risk factors these populations [40].

Acknowledgment

The author expresses gratitude to Dr. Terry A. Lennie for his assistance with the preparation of this article.

References

[1] Rosamond W, Flegal K, Friday G, et al. Heart disease and stroke statistics—2007 Update. A report from the American Heart Association Statistics Committee and Stroke Statistics Subcommittee. Circulation 2007;115:E69–171.

[2] De Caterina R, Zampolli A, Del Turco S, et al. Nutritional mechanisms that influence cardiovascular disease. Am J Clin Nutr 2006;83(2):421S–6S.

[3] Giugliano D, Ceriello A, Esposito K. The effects of diet on inflammation: emphasis on the metabolic syndrome. J Am Coll Cardiol 2006;48(4):677–85.

[4] Schulz AJ, Kannan S, Dvonch JT, et al. Social and physical environments and disparities in risk for cardiovascular disease: the healthy environments partnership conceptual model. Environ Health Perspect 2005;113(12):1817–25.

[5] Trichopoulou A, Lagiou P. Healthy traditional Mediterranean diet: an expression of culture, history and lifestyle. Nutr Rev 1997;55:383–9.

[6] Chrysohoou C, Panagiotakos D, Pitsavos C, et al. Adherence to the Mediterranean diet attenuates inflammation and coagulation process in healthy adults: the ATTICA Study. J Am Coll Cardiol 2004;44(1):152–8.

[7] Esposito K, Marfella R, Ciotola M, et al. Effect of a Mediterranean-style diet on endothelial dysfunction and markers of vascular inflammation in the metabolic syndrome. JAMA 2004; 292(12):1440–6.

[8] Zarraga IGE, Schwarz ER. Impact of dietary patterns and interventions on cardiovascular health. Circulation 2006;114(9):961–73.

[9] Davis N, Katz S, Wylie-Rosett J. The effect of diet on endothelial function. Cardiol Rev 2007;15(2):62–6.

[10] National Cholesterol Education Program (NCEP). Third report of the expert panel on detection, evaluation, and treatment of high blood cholesterol in adults (Adult Treatment Panel III). NIH Publication No. 02-5215. Bethesda (MD): National Institutes of Health, National Heart, Lung, and Blood Institute; 2002.

[11] Gropper SS, Smith JL, Groff JL. Lipids. In: Howe E, Feldman E, editors. Advanced nutrition and human metabolism. 4th edition. Belmont (CA): Thomson Wadsworth; 2005. p. 146–7, 157–159.

[12] De Lorgeril M, Renaud S, Mamelle N, et al. Mediterranean alpha-linolenic acid rich-diet in secondary prevention of coronary heart disease. Lancet 1994;343:1454–9.

[13] Simopoulos AP. Evolutionary aspects of diet, the omega-6/omega-3 ratio and genetic variation: nutritional implications for chronic diseases. Biomed Pharmacother 2006;60(9): 502–7.

[14] Schwalfenberg G. Omega-3 fatty acids: their beneficial role in cardiovascular health. Can Fam Physician 2006;52:734–40.

[15] Chrysohoou C, Panagiotakos DB, Pitsavos C, et al. Long-term fish consumption is associated with protection against arrhythmia in healthy persons in a Mediterranean region- the ATTICA study. Am J Clin Nutr 2007;85(5):1385–91.

[16] West SG, Hecker KD, Mustad VA, et al. Acute effects of monounsaturated fatty acids with and without omega-3 fatty acids on vascular reactivity in individuals with type 2 diabetes. Diabetologia 2005;48:113–22.

[17] Erkkila AT, Matthan NR, Herrington DM, et al. Higher plasma docosahexaenoic acid is associated with reduced progression of coronary atherosclerosis in women with CAD. J Lipid Res 2006;47:2814–9.

[18] Morgan DR, Dixon LJ, Hanratty CG, et al. Effects of dietary omega-3 fatty acid supplementation on endothelium-dependent vasodilation in patients with chronic heart failure. Am J Cardiol 2006;97(4):547–51.

[19] Huang PH, Chen JW, Lu TM, et al. Combined use of endothelial function assessed by brachial ultrasound and high-sensitive C-reactive protein in predicting cardiovascular events. Clin Cardiol 2007;30(3):135–40.

[20] Harris WS, Reid KJ, Sands SA, et al. Blood omega-3 and trans fatty acids in middle-aged acute coronary syndrome patients. Am J Cardiol 2007;99(2):154–8.

[21] Cao J, Schwichtenberg KA, Hanson NA, et al. Incorporation and clearance of omega-3 fatty acids in erythrocyte membranes and plasma phospholipids. Clin Chem 2006;52: 2265–72.

[22] Mozaffarian D. Does alpha-linolenic acid intake reduce the risk of coronary heart disease? A review of the evidence. Altern Ther Health Med 2005;11(3):24–30.

[23] Perona J, Cabello-Moruno R, Ruiz-Gutierrez V. The role of virgin olive oil in the modulation of endothelial function. J Nutr Biochem 2005;17(7):429–45.

[24] Dauchet L, Amouyel P, Hercberg S, et al. Fruit and vegetable consumption and risk of coronary heart disease: a meta-analysis of cohort studies. J Nutr 2006;136:2588–93.

[25] Yoon J, Baek SJ. Molecular targets of dietary polyphenols with anti-inflammatory properties. Yonsei Med J 2005;46(5):585–96.

[26] Zern TL, Fernandez ML. Cardioprotective effects of dietary polyphenols. J Nutr 2005;135: 2291–4.

[27] Chun OK, Chung SJ, Song WO. Estimated dietary flavonoid intake and major foods sources of U.S. adults. J Nutr 2007;137:1244–52.

[28] Gropper SS, Smith JL, Groff JL. The fat-soluble vitamins. In: Howe E, Feldman E, editors. Advanced nutrition and human metabolism. 4th edition. Belmont (CA): Thomson Wadsworth; 2005. p. 352–9, 371–6.

[29] Lapointe A, Couillard C, Lemieux S. Effects of dietary factors on oxidation of low-density lipoprotein particles. J Nutr Biochem 2006;17:645–58.

[30] Mead A, Atkinson G, Albin D, et al. Dietetic guidelines on food and nutrition in the secondary prevention of cardiovascular disease—evidence from systematic reviews of randomized controlled trials. J Hum Nutr Diet 2006;19:401–19.

[31] Riccioni G, Bucciarelli T, Mancini B, et al. The role of the antioxidant vitamin supplementation in the prevention of cardiovascular diseases. Expert Opin Investig Drugs 2007;16(1): 25–32.

[32] Carlsson C. Homocysteine lowering with folic acid and vitamin B supplements: effects on cardiovascular disease in older adults. Drugs Aging 2006;23(6):491–502.

[33] Gropper SS, Smith JL, Groff JL. The water-soluble vitamins. In: Howe E, Feldman E, editors. Advanced nutrition and human metabolism. 4th edition. Belmont (CA): Thomson Wadsworth; 2005. p. 301–9.

[34] Gropper SS, Smith JL, Groff JL. Fiber. In: Advanced nutrition and human metabolism. 4th edition. Belmont (CA): Thomson Wadsworth; 2005. p. 115–9.

[35] Salas-Salvado J, Garcia-Arellano A, Estruch R, et al. Components of the Mediterranean-type food pattern and serum inflammatory markers among patients at high risk for cardiovascular disease. Eur J Clin Nutr 2007; doi:10.1038/sj.ejcn. 1602762.

[36] Vasdev S, Gill V, Singal PK. Beneficial effect of low ethanol intake on the cardiovascular system: possible biochemical mechanisms. Vasc Health Risk Manag 2006;2(3):263–76.

[37] Simopoulous AP. The Mediterranean diets: what is so special about the diet of Greece? The scientific evidence. J Nutr 2001;131:3065S–73S.

[38] Pruett BS, Pruett SB. An explanation for the paradoxical induction and suppression of an acute phase response by ethanol. Alcohol 2006;39(2):105–10.

[39] Ellison RC, Zhang Y, Qureshi MM, et al. Lifestyle determinants of high-density lipoprotein cholesterol: the National Heart, Lung, and Blood Institute Family Heart Study. Am Heart J 2004;147(3):529–35.

[40] Tessaro I, Rye S, Parker L, et al. Effectiveness of a nutrition intervention with rural low-income women. Am J Health Behav 2007;31(1):35–43.

ELSEVIER
SAUNDERS

Nurs Clin N Am 43 (2008) 117–132

NURSING
CLINICS
OF NORTH AMERICA

Nutritional Considerations in Heart Failure

Heather Payne-Emerson, BS, RD[a],*,
Terry A. Lennie, PhD, RN[a,b]

[a]Graduate Center for Nutritional Sciences, University of Kentucky, Lexington, KY, USA
[b]College of Nursing, University of Kentucky,
760 Rose Street, Lexington, KY 40536-0232, USA

Current heart failure (HF) guidelines provide only a few recommendations for the nutritional management of patients who have HF [1,2]. This is primarily because of the limited research available for establishing evidence-based recommendations. This article reviews the available information regarding sodium, fluid restriction, and other nutritional recommendations to assist clinicians in nutritional management of patients who have HF.

This information on other nutritional recommendations is reviewed in the context of our current understanding of several potential interactions among nutrients, HF pathophysiology, and treatment. First, inflammation is recognized to play an important role in HF pathophysiology [3–6]. Elevated levels of proinflammatory cytokines may lead to the development of cardiac cachexia [7,8] as well as promote progression of HF [5]. Nutritional intake, particularly dietary fat, may modulate the inflammatory process. Second, it has been demonstrated that oxidative stress is present at increased levels in HF [9]. Certain micronutrients have antioxidant capabilities [10–12] and influence vascular and cardiac function [13–18]. Diuretic use may increase excretion of these nutrients [13,19], indicating a need to assure adequate micronutrient intake. Third, the recent evidence suggesting that increased body fat is related to better outcomes in HF has nutritional implications regarding recommending weight loss in overweight and obese patients [20–24]. Fourth, many patients have comorbidities that require dietary modifications [25–27]. These modifications need to be considered when assisting patients with nutritional management of HF.

* Corresponding author.
  E-mail address: hmpayn2@uky.edu (H. Payne-Emerson).

0029-6465/08/$ - see front matter © 2008 Elsevier Inc. All rights reserved.
doi:10.1016/j.cnur.2007.10.003
nursing.theclinics.com

Sodium

Dietary sodium restriction is recommended by the American College of Cardiology/American Heart Association (ACC/AHA) [2] and Heart Failure Society of America (HFSA) [1], but is only suggested in the European Society of Cardiology (ESC) [28,29] HF guidelines. The primary evidence cited to support these recommendations is professional opinion. Although some studies have found that HF maintenance programs involving diet education decrease the number of hospital readmissions [30–33], the results cannot be solely attributed to alterations in the diet.

Currently, there is no consensus among the guidelines regarding the suggested level of restriction. The HFSA guidelines recommend a 2 to 3 g sodium restriction for less advanced stages of HF, and less than 2 g for moderate to severe HF [1]. The ACC/AHA guidelines call for sodium restriction of 2 g only for those who have end-stage HF. Patients who have less severe HF have a more liberal 3 to 4 g restriction [2]. The ESC makes no specific recommendation, but rather suggests that patients who have severe HF may benefit from limiting sodium intake [28,29]. In contrast, the 2005 United States Department of Agriculture Dietary Guidelines for Americans [34] and the AHA Nutrition Committee 2006 Diet and Lifestyle Recommendations [35] both suggest sodium restriction of less than 2.3 g for all healthy Americans. The logic of recommending a limit that is higher than in healthy individuals is questionable.

Regardless, there is a consensus among the three guidelines that excess sodium intake may exacerbate symptoms of HF by causing fluid retention [1,2,28,29], and that restricting sodium intake may allow for a lower diuretic dose [1,2]. Randomized controlled clinical trials may provide the evidence needed to support a specific level of sodium restriction. In the meantime, there is no evidence of harm related to sodium restriction; therefore working with patients to achieve a level of sodium intake between 2 to 3 g seems a reasonable compromise among all guidelines.

Fluid

Current guidelines include a recommended fluid restriction of 1.5 [29] to 2 [1,2,29] L per day in patients with advanced HF or persistent fluid retention with high diuretic dose [1,2]. Again, evidence to support these recommendations is clinical expertise as there were no clinical trials available. One, randomized, controlled study was recently published. Travers and colleagues [36] reported 1 L fluid restriction had no benefit over no fluid restriction with respect to time to clinical stability in NYHA Class IV hospitalized patients. There were also no differences in diuretic dose, daily fluid output, or average weight loss from baseline to clinical stability. Interestingly, the unrestricted group consumed an average of only 1466 ($\pm$607) mL. This suggests that patients were spontaneously consuming a low amount of fluid, and that it may not be necessary for clinicians to enforce fluid restriction; however, the observation also suggests that this study was not a test of whether fluid restriction in patients who spontaneously consume higher amounts of fluid would be beneficial. Further research is needed to clarify the issue. In the meantime, clinicians may wish to observe patients spontaneous fluid intake before imposing what may be unnecessary measures to restrict fluids.

Inflammation and cachexia

Heart failure is considered an inflammatory condition that is marked by elevated proinflammatory cytokine activity, particularly interleukin (IL)-6 and tumor necrosis factor-alpha (TNFα) [3–6]. Inflammation is believed to contribute to the progression of HF by contributing to cardiac remodeling and suppression of myocardial function [5,37]. It is also believed to play a role in the development of cachexia, an independent risk factor for mortality in HF [38], by promoting tissue catabolism and decreasing appetite [39].

The HFSA guidelines recommend caloric supplementation for the nutritional management of cardiac cachexia [1]. The assessment of nitrogen balance, prealbumin, and caloric intake are recommended indicators for the determination of appropriate supplementation. Consideration of formal metabolic evaluation and determination of minimum nutritional requirements are also suggested. Although no clinical trial data are available, ESC guidelines recommend small, frequent, high energy meals to maximize caloric intake in the presence of anorexia [29]. This is clearly an area where additional research is needed.

Dietary fats

There is evidence that changes to patient diets, particularly dietary fats, may decrease the level of inflammation [40,41] and subsequently cachexia. Inflammatory cytokines are activated by cell membrane-derived ecosanoids that are synthesized from omega-6 (n-6) fatty acids in the lipid component of cell membranes [42,43]. In contrast, ecosanoids synthesized from omega-3 (n-3) fatty acids are more immunoneutral [44]. The n-3 fatty acids, particularly eicosapentaenoic acid (EPA) and docosahexaenoic acid (DHA), can competitively inhibit the incorporation of n-6 fatty acids into cell membranes [42,43], and thus can lead to a decrease in n-6 derived ecosanoids when consumed in adequate amounts [43]. Therefore, it seems logical that increased consumption of n-3 fatty acids could reduce the production of proinflammatory cytokines and potentially aid in the treatment of cachexia and limit progression of HF.

Although limited, the data available regarding the effect of n-3 fatty acids in HF suggest a potential benefit. In a placebo-controlled study using a canine model of HF [45], a significant improvement in cardiac cachexia and decrease in the levels of proinflammatory cytokine IL-1 were observed after supplementation with fish oil. In a small randomized, double-blind, placebo-controlled trial, patients were provided a supplementation of 8 g of n-3 fatty acids. The sample consisted of 14 patients at New York Heart Association (NYHA) Classes III and IV, 57% of whom had cachexia. The researchers found a 59% decrease of in vitro TNFα production in the supplemented group. There was a significant difference in the change in body fat between the treatment and placebo group (+13% verses −5%, respectively); however, no significant changes were seen in body weight, indicating that lean body mass (LBM) did not improve [46].

There is one study in which the effects of the composition of fats in the diets of community-dwelling patients who had HF was examined [47]. Patients consuming higher amounts of saturated and trans fats were found to have significantly higher levels of TNFα in their blood. In contrast, patients consuming higher amounts of n-3 fatty acids had lower blood levels of inflammatory markers. These patients also had significantly better event-free (hospitalization or death) survival than those who had higher blood levels of inflammatory markers. This suggests that the composition of fats in the diet can affect outcomes by altering the severity of inflammation. These results are similar to a study of 859 healthy adults in which participants who had higher intakes of EPA and DHA had significantly lower levels of soluble TNF receptors (markers in inflammatory activity) [48]. This association, however, was only found in people who also had a high n-6 fatty acid intake. This makes intuitive sense because n-3 fatty acids would only be expected to make a competitive difference in the cell membranes of people who have diets that also contain excessive amounts of proinflammatory n-6 fatty acids. Supporting this assumption are studies in which adults fed experimental diets containing trans [49,50] and saturated fat [49] showed significantly higher levels of TNFα, IL-6, [49] and C-reactive protein (CRP) [50] after consumption.

There is a growing body of evidence supporting the benefits of n-3 fatty acids on cardiovascular disease (CVD) [51] suggesting that adequate intake of n-3s may be advisable for patients who have HF, regardless of the presence of cachexia. Possible mechanisms include hypotriglyceridemic effects, mild hypotensive effects, decreased platelet aggregation, decreased progression of atherosclerotic plaque (including anti-inflammatory effects), and antiarrhythmic effects. The AHA recommends that patients who have CVD consume a combined total of 1 g of EPA and DHA per day, which can most easily be obtained from fatty fish. Fish oil supplements are recognized as an alternative for those who do not consume fish or if contaminated fish are a concern [51].

Mediterranean diet

The Mediterranean diet has also been proposed as a means to decrease inflammation, although no studies in HF have been conducted. This diet is rich in fruits, vegetables, nuts, whole grains, poultry, and fish, with moderate consumption of wine (1 to 2 glasses per day), and olive oil as the primary lipid. Additionally, red meats are consumed rarely, and sweets are consumed only on a weekly basis [52]. Participants in the Attica Study who most closely adhered to the Mediterranean diet had significantly lower levels of CRP, IL-6, and fibrinogen (20%, 17%, and 6% respectively), even after controlling for age, gender, smoking, physical activity, financial status, body mass index (BMI), hypertension, diabetes, hypercholesterolemia, and family history of CVD [53]. Esposito and colleagues [54] studied the effects of the Mediterranean diet in individuals who had metabolic syndrome. Participants who consumed a Mediterranean diet as instructed had significantly decreased levels of IL-6, IL-7, IL-18, and high-sensitivity CRP after 2 years compared with the control group who consumed a prudent diet with the same macronutrient distribution. Although these studies did not include patients who had HF, the evidence does suggest that the Mediterranean diet, other diets lower in saturated and trans fats, and diets with a lower ratio of n-6 to n-3 fatty acids may decrease inflammation in patients who have HF.

Protein and caloric intake

Protein is an essential macronutrient involved in the composition and maintenance of body structure, muscles, and enzymes, as well as body transport, regulatory, and immune systems [55]. There are data to suggest that certain amino acids may aid in the treatment of cachexia. Combinations of β-hydroxy-β-methylbutyrate (a leucine metabolite), arginine, and glutamine have been shown to increase lean body mass in other forms of cachexia such as cancer [56] and AIDS-associated wasting [57]. The observation that branch chain amino acid supplementation could decrease muscle loss associated with extended bed rest has led to speculation that these amino acids could potentially aid in the treatment of cachexia [58]; however, more evidence is needed to support amino acid supplementation in HF.

The HFSA guidelines recommend that patients who have HF consume a level of protein appropriate for their age, gender, and activity level [1]. No other recommendations for protein intake in HF are available. The dietary reference intake for protein in healthy adults is 0.8 g/kg body weight per day; however, disease states can increase the body's demand for protein and increase protein turnover [59]. Thus, it is reasonable to suspect that protein requirements could be higher in this population. A study by Aquilani and colleagues [60] found that 60% of patients who had HF had a negative nitrogen balance, despite consuming a similar amount of protein (approximately 1 g/kg) as a healthy age- and BMI-matched group. Similarly, patients had comparable calorie intake, but had significantly higher energy expenditure. Thus, it is not surprising that 70% of these patients had a negative energy balance. It should be noted that protein can be used for energy if caloric intake is inadequate [59]. Therefore, although the negative nitrogen balance indicates that patients had increased protein turnover, this could also be caused by protein being used to meet increased energy requirements. Regardless, the data suggest that patients who have HF may benefit from diets higher in protein and calories than healthy adults.

Micronutrients

As is the case with sodium restriction, there is no consensus among the major guidelines regarding micronutrient supplementation in patients who have HF. ACC/AHA guidelines acknowledge that patients taking diuretics may become deficient in some micronutrients [2]; however, supplementation to correct these deficiencies is not recommended because no benefit has been demonstrated. Conversely, the HFSA guidelines support the use of a daily multivitamin and mineral supplement to combat effects of early satiety, decreased absorption of nutrients, and loss of water-soluble vitamins and minerals caused by diuretic use [1].

There is evidence that patients who have HF are at risk for micronutrient deficiencies. Gorelik and colleagues [61] found through 6-month diet recall that patients who had HF had lower than recommended intake of magnesium, calcium, zinc, copper, manganese, thiamine, riboflavin, and folate; however, low intake of these nutrients was also found in a group of patients free of HF. This finding is understandable, considering that the study was conducted in hospitalized adults over 60 years old who may have experienced barriers to adequate intake before hospitalization [62].

The benefits of micronutrient supplementation have been demonstrated in a small randomized, double-blind, placebo-controlled trial by Witte and colleagues [63]. This group found improved quality of life, increased left ventricular ejection fraction, and decreased left ventricular volume in patients taking a high doses of several vitamins and minerals compared with patients receiving a placebo. Food intake was not measured, so it is not known if patients who had nutrient deficiencies benefited more than patients who had adequate nutritional intake.

Magnesium

Magnesium is an essential mineral that is a cofactor in multiple enzyme systems in the body. It plays a role in nucleotide synthesis, intracellular potassium maintenance, and as a natural calcium channel blocker [13]. Magnesium deficiency can result in cardiac arrhythmias [13]. Deficient intake of magnesium has been found in patients who have HF [61,64]. Additionally, diuretics use may contribute to magnesium deficiency by promoting urinary loss [13,65]. Thus, magnesium supplementation may be beneficial.

Calcium

Calcium is a principal component of teeth and bones, but it also plays a role in vasodilation, and in vascular and muscle contractility. Chronic deficiencies in calcium intake lead to osteopenia and osteoporosis [14], and may contribute to cardiac dysrhythmias [15]. Diets of patients who have HF have been documented to be deficient in calcium [61]. Intestinal calcium absorption declines with age, and subsequently the established adequate intake for adults over the age of 50 increases from 1000 mg to 1200 mg. Further, loop diuretics increase excretion of calcium [19]. Additionally, vitamin D is essential for the absorption of calcium [14], which has also been found to be deficient in diets of many patients [66]. Thus, patients who have HF, especially older patients, may benefit from combined calcium and vitamin D supplementation.

Vitamin D

Vitamin D is a fat-soluble vitamin whose only major function was originally thought to be maintenance of calcium and phosphorus blood levels by stimulating intestinal absorption of these minerals [67]. A recent review summarized the results of several studies assessing vitamin D status in patients who had HF [68]. In the majority of these studies, mean serum 25-hydroxy vitamin D concentrations were in the insufficient range, although the standard deviations were quite large, indicating a wide range of vitamin D levels in patients. Another study indicated that patients who have HF have lower circulating levels of 25-hydroxy vitamin D compared with age-matched case controls [69]. Vitamin D insufficiency may play a role in the development of CVD and hypertension through regulation of both parathyroid hormone and the renin-angiotensin system, and through its influence on myocardial cell proliferation [68] and myocardial hypertrophy [68,70]. Lower levels of 25-hydroxy vitamin D have also been associated with increased severity of HF. Thus, vitamin D insufficiency may contribute to the pathogenesis of HF.

There may be other roles for vitamin D including influencing cardiac contractility [16] and production of proinflammatory cytokines [71]. Schleithoff and colleagues [71] conducted a randomized, double-blind, placebo-controlled trial to assess the effect of vitamin D supplementation on cytokine levels in patients who had HF. Ninety-three men who had HF were randomized into two groups, one receiving 2000 IU of cholecalciferol with 500 mg of calcium, the other a placebo and 500 mg calcium for 9 months. Although no significant differences were seen in survival during the 15-month follow-up period, the vitamin D group had significantly higher levels of the anti-inflammatory cytokine IL-10 compared with baseline values, whereas the placebo group had no change. TNFα levels did not change in the vitamin D supplemented group compared with baseline values, but were significantly increased in the placebo group compared with baseline. This suggests that the vitamin D-supplemented group had a beneficial shift in the ratio of anti-inflammatory to proinflammatory cytokines.

In vitro and animal studies in other disease states involving inflammation have demonstrated that vitamin D and its analogs inhibit TNFα [72], and in conjunction with calcium also down-regulate TNFα gene expression [73]. Incubation of cells in the presence of vitamin D or its analogs has also decreased the production of IL-6 [74] and IL-8 [75]. It is important to note that although the vitamin D analogs used in these studies were designed to prevent high-dose toxic effects, the amount of naturally occurring vitamin D necessary to elicit the observed response is well above levels considered safe for human consumption.

In sum, the evidence suggests that prevention of vitamin D deficiency may provide additional benefits beyond those traditionally associated with this vitamin. Adequate intake of vitamin D is important to maintain normal physiological functioning, regardless of the additional benefits it may or may not have.

Selenium

A major function of selenium is protection against oxidative stress [10], which has been demonstrated to be high in HF [9]. Selenium deficiency leads to decreased activity of antioxidant enzymes, and is compounded by a concurrent deficiency in vitamin E [10], another important antioxidant [11]. It is suspected that low selenium levels compromise cardiovascular function and influence clinical severity of HF because of its important role in antioxidant systems. Additionally, maximally improved exercise capacity has been demonstrated with selenium intakes of 80 µg per day, a level much higher than the current recommendation of 55 to 70 µg per day [76]. Thus, supplementation may be beneficial, especially in geographic areas in which naturally occurring selenium in the soil is low.

Vitamin E

Vitamin E is a fat-soluble vitamin with important antioxidant abilities [11]; however, the benefit of vitamin E supplementation in HF is debatable. A randomized, placebo-controlled study demonstrated no benefit of vitamin E supplementation on indices of oxidative stress, quality of life, natriuretic peptide, or proinflammatory cytokine levels [77]. Vitamin E supplementation may even increase development of and hospitalization for HF [78], as well as mortality risk [79,80]. In sum, vitamin E is an essential and safe nutrient when obtained from food, but caution should be used with supplements.

Thiamin

Thiamin acts as a coenzyme for carbohydrate and branched-chain amino acid metabolism. Deficiencies of this water-soluble vitamin lead to anorexia, weight loss, muscle weakness, myocardial hypertrophy [17], myocardial failure, and sodium and water retention [18]. Long-term diuretic use [18,81,82], malnutrition, advanced age, severe HF, and frequent hospitalizations have all been associated with thiamin deficiency in patients who have HF [82].

Estimates of the incidence of thiamin deficiency in patients who have HF ranges from 13% to 93% [82]. This suggests that supplementation may be beneficial.

Folate and vitamin B12

Homocysteine is an amino acid that is thought to promote atherosclerosis through several mechanisms, including injury to vascular endothelium and increased oxidative stress. Folate and B_{12} are essential for the conversion of homocysteine to methionine [15], and an inverse relationship exists between intakes of these vitamins and homocysteine levels [65]. Elevated levels of homocysteine are associated with HF [76], and recent evidence suggests that homocysteine is also related to clinical severity [83,84] and mortality [83] in HF. Although the presence of hyperhomocysteinemia in HF is not necessarily only caused by deficiencies of folate and B_{12}, the possibility of lowering homocysteine via supplementation of these vitamins is intriguing. Deficiencies of B_{12} are of particular concern in older patients. Older adults tend to have decreased plasma levels of B_{12}, a condition indicative of decreased vitamin B_{12} status. This is potentially because of the higher prevalence of atrophic gastritis in the elderly. This leads to decreased stomach acid and intrinsic factor secretion, two factors necessary for the absorption of B_{12} [85]. In these patients, alternative routes of B_{12} supplementation may be required.

Vitamin C

Vitamin C is an important water-soluble vitamin because of its substantial antioxidant properties. Additionally, it promotes regeneration of the antioxidant activity of vitamin E [12]. There are many beneficial cardiovascular-related effects of vitamin C in HF, including improved endothelial function and decreased cardiomyocyte and endothelial apoptosis [65]. Although there are limited data, deficiencies of vitamin C have been found in patients who have HF [65]. Given that vitamin C is water soluble, adequate daily intake is important.

Obesity

Obesity is associated with increased risk for the development of HF [86]. Current guidelines by the HFSA [1] and ESC [29] recommend weight loss for obese patients who have HF as a means of improving prognosis; however, the only evidence used to support this recommendation is a study by Alpert and colleagues [87] that showed improvements in NYHA functional class after gastroplasty induced weight loss in morbidly obese patients. A number of studies have demonstrated an association between higher BMI and improved outcomes in HF [20–23], even when patients who have cachexia are excluded [21,22]. One suggested mechanism for this association is differing cytokine profiles in obese patients [20]. There is evidence that soluble TNF receptors 1 and 2 positively correlate with BMI [24], and these receptors have also been shown to have inhibitory effects on their proinflammatory ligand, TNF-α [88]. A positive correlation between IL-6 and BMI has also been demonstrated [24]. Although IL-6 is a proinflammatory cytokine, it is acknowledged to have anti-inflammatory effects as well [89]. It has been postulated that these anti-inflammatory actions in obese patients who have HF may provide a protective effect [90].

An alternative reason for better outcomes in obese patients is that patients included in some of the studies were incorrectly diagnosed with HF because of the presence of dyspnea and edema [91]; however, patients in several studies were referred for evaluation for transplant, and therefore were not likely to be misdiagnosed [20,21]. Others have suggested that obese patients may present at an earlier and less severe level of HF, and thus appear to have a better prognosis [92]. More research is needed to clarify this paradox and determine if the relationship found in previous studies is causal or an epiphenomenon. In the meantime, decisions to recommend weight loss should be made on an individual basis.

Comorbidities

Arteriosclerosis

Current HFSA guidelines [1] recommend that patients who have HF and arteriosclerosis or hyperlipidemia receive dietary instruction based on guidelines such as those of the National Cholesterol Education Program [25]. These guidelines suggest implementing the Therapeutic Lifestyle Changes (TLC) diet, which emphasizes reducing saturated fat intake to less than 7% of total calories and cholesterol to less than 200 mg per day. These recommendations are also incorporated into the American Diabetes Association (ADA) guidelines [26] and the Dietary Approaches to Stop Hypertension (DASH) guidelines [27] discussed later. The TLC diet also includes specific recommendations for macronutrient distribution, fiber intake, and the use of plant stanols and sterols to aid in the reduction of LDL levels [25].

Diabetes

Diabetes mellitus (DM) is considered a major risk factor in the development of HF [2]. Furthermore, DM increases the risk of hospital readmission [93,94] and mortality in patients who have HF [94], and the progression of HF may be quickened by hyperinsulinemia, via promotion of cardiac and vascular hypertrophy [2].

Although the ESC guidelines [29] do not include recommendations concerning DM, both the ACC/AHA [2] and HFSA [1] guidelines include a recommendation for standard treatment (ie, tight control of blood glucose) of

DM regardless of the presence of HF. The HFSA guidelines also encourage individualized counseling regarding appropriate carbohydrate, protein, and calorie intake [1]. This is in line with the current ADA guidelines, which emphasize that medical nutrition therapy be provided by a registered dietitian. Principally, carbohydrate intake should be closely monitored using exchange or carbohydrate counting methods. A diet rich in fruits, vegetables, low-fat and fat-free dairy products, whole grains, fiber, and legumes is encouraged, which is similar to a modified Mediterranean style diet. Patients are advised to limit saturated fat to less than 7% of total calories, minimize trans fat, consume two servings a week of n-3 fatty acid-containing fish, decrease sodium intake, and consume no more than 200 mg of dietary cholesterol/day [26].

These guidelines are slightly more restrictive than the USDA Dietary Guidelines, which suggest that healthy adults should keep saturated fat and cholesterol intake to less than 10% and 300 mg/day respectively [34]; however, the ADA recommendations for saturated fat and cholesterol mirror those made by the National Cholesterol Education Program, which were designed to lower LDL in those at risk for CVD [25].

Hypertension

Hypertension (HTN) is also considered a risk factor for developing HF, and may hasten the progression of those who have HF [2]. The DASH diet was designed to provide rich sources of fiber, potassium, magnesium, calcium, and protein as a means of treating HTN [27]. The basic principles of this diet are in accordance with the ADA guidelines for DM and the US Department of Agriculture (USDA) Dietary Guidelines for Americans, with the emphasis on whole grains, fruits, vegetables, low-fat or fat-free dairy products, lean meats, and legumes. The number of servings recommended for each food group is based on calorie level, with high intakes of fruits, vegetables, and grains [27,34].

Discussion

The principals underlying the dietary recommendations for all three common comorbidities are consistent with those for managing HF independent of comorbidities. Thus, none of these diets conflict with HF management goals. Although it is possible for a patient to incorporate recommendations from all three diets, careful planning with a registered dietitian will most likely be required.

Summary

Catabolism, inflammation, oxidative stress, diuretic use, and comorbidities may alter the nutritional needs of patients who have HF. Intake of some nutrients may need to be increased to meet changing demands, whereas others have been suggested as modulators of disease processes. Additional research is needed to define specific micro- and macronutrient ranges for this population, as well as to provide evidence regarding the longstanding recommendations of sodium and fluid restriction.

References

[1] Adams KF, Arnold JMO, Baker DW, et al. HFSA 2006 comprehensive heart failure practice guidelines. J Card Fail 2006;12:e29–37.

[2] Hunt SA. ACC/AHA 2005 guideline update for the diagnosis and management of chronic heart failure in the adult: a report of the American College of Cardiology/American Heart Association Task Force on Practice Guidelines (Writing Committee to Update the 2001 Guidelines for the Evaluation and Management of Heart Failure). J Am Coll Cardiol 2005;46(6):e1–e82.

[3] Munger MA, Johnson B, Amber IJ, et al. Circulating concentrations of proinflammatory cytolcines in mild or moderate heart failure secondary to ischemic or idiopathic dilated cardiomyopathy. Am J Cardiol 1996;77(9):723–7.

[4] Aukrust P, Ueland T, Lien E, et al. Cytokine network in congestive heart failure secondary to ischemic or idiopathic dilated cardiomyopathy. J Am Coll Cardiol 1999;83(3):376–82.

[5] Conraads VM, Bosmans JM, Vrints CJ. Chronic heart failure: an example of a systemic chronic inflammatory disease resulting in cachexia. Int J Cardiol 2002;85(1):33–49.

[6] Milani RV, Mehra MR, Endres S, et al. The clinical relevance of circulating tumor necrosis factor-alpha in acute decompensated chronic heart failure without cachexia. Chest 1996;110(4):992–5.

[7] Filippatos GS, Anker SD, Kremastinos DT. Pathophysiology of peripheral muscle wasting in cardiac cachexia. Curr Opin Clin Nutr Metab Care 2005;8(3):249–54.

[8] von Haehling S, Doehner W, Anker SD. Nutrition, metabolism, and the complex pathophysiology of cachexia in chronic heart failure. Cardiovasc Res 2007;73(2):298–309.

[9] MacCarthy PA, Shah AM. Oxidative stress and heart failure. Coron Artery Dis 2003;14(2):109–13.

[10] Institute of Medicine. Selenium. dietary reference intakes for vitamin C, vitamin E, selenium and carotenoids. Washington, DC: National Academy Press; 2000. p. 284–324.

[11] Institute of Medicine. Vitamin E. Dietary reference intakes for vitamin c, vitamin e, selenium and carotenoids. Washington, DC: National Academy Press; 2000. p. 186–283.

[12] Institute of Medicine. Vitamin C. Dietary reference intakes for vitamin C, vitamin E, selenium and carotenoids. Washington, DC: National Academy Press; 2000. p. 95–185.

[13] Institute of Medicine. Magnesium. Dietary reference intakes for calcium, phosphorus, magnesium, vitamin D and fluoride. Washington, D.C: National Academy Press; 1997. p. 190–249.

[14] Institute of Medicine. Calcium. Dietary reference intakes for calcium, phosphorus, magnesium, vitamin D and fluoride. Washington, DC: National Academy Press; 1997. p. 71–145.

[15] Witte KK, Clark AL, Cleland JG. Chronic heart failure and micronutrients. J Am Coll Cardiol 2001;37(7):1765–74.

[16] Green JJ, Robinson DA, Wilson GE, et al. Calcitriol modulation of cardiac contractile performance via protein kinase C. J Mol Cell Cardiol 2006;41(2):350–9.

[17] Institute of Medicine. Thiamin. Dietary reference intakes for thiamin, riboflavin, niacin, vitamin B6, folate, vitamin B12, pantothenic acid, biotin, and choline. Washington, DC: National Academy Press; 1998. p. 58–86.

[18] Leslie D, Gheorghiade M. Is there a role for thiamine supplementation in the management of heart failure? Am Heart J 1996;131(6):1248–50.

[19] Stier CT Jr, Itskovitz HD. Renal calcium metabolism and diuretics. Annu Rev Pharmacol Toxicol 1986;26:101–16.

[20] Horwich TB, Fonarow GC, Hamilton MA, et al. The relationship between obesity and mortality in patients with heart failure. J Am Coll Cardiol 2001;38(3):789–95.

[21] Lavie CJ, Osman AF, Milani RV, et al. Body composition and prognosis in chronic systolic heart failure: the obesity paradox. Am J Cardiol 2003;91(7):891–4.

[22] Bozkurt B, Deswal A. Obesity as a prognostic factor in chronic symptomatic heart failure. Am Heart J 2005;150(6):1233–9.

[23] Mosterd A, Cost B, Hoes AW, et al. The prognosis of heart failure in the general population. The Rotterdam Study. Eur Heart J 2001;22(15):1318–27.

[24] Mohamed-Ali V, Goodrick S, Bulmer K, et al. Production of soluble tumor necrosis factor receptors by human subcutaneous adipose tissue in vivo. Am J Physiol 1999;277(6 Pt 1): E971–5.

[25] Executive summary of the third report of the National Cholesterol Education Program (NCEP) expert panel on detection, evaluation, and treatment of high blood cholesterol in adults (Adult Treatment Panel III). JAMA 2001;285(19):2486–97.

[26] Bantle JP, Wylie-Rosett J, Albright AL, et al. Nutrition recommendations and interventions for diabetes—2006: a position statement of the American Diabetes Association. Diabetes Care 2006;29(9):2140–57.

[27] Appel LJ, Moore TJ, Obarzanek E, et al. A clinical trial of the effects of dietary patterns on blood pressure. DASH Collaborative Research Group. N Engl J Med 1997;336(16):1117–24.

[28] Swedberg K, Cleland J, Dargie H, et al. Guidelines for the diagnosis and treatment of chronic heart failure: executive summary (update 2005): The Task Force for the Diagnosis and Treatment of Chronic Heart Failure of the European Society of Cardiology. Eur Heart J 2005; 26(11):1115–40.

[29] Guidelines for the diagnosis and treatment of chronic heart failure. 2005. Available at: http://escardio.org. Accessed September 3, 2007.

[30] Rich MW, Beckham V, Wittenberg C, et al. A multidisciplinary intervention to prevent the readmission of elderly patients with congestive heart failure. N Engl J Med 1995;333(18): 1190–5.

[31] Shah NB, Der E, Ruggerio C, et al. Prevention of hospitalizations for heart failure with an interactive home monitoring program. Am Heart J 1998;135(3):373–8.

[32] Fonarow GC, Stevenson LW, Walden JA, et al. Impact of a comprehensive heart failure management program on hospital readmission and functional status of patients with advanced heart failure. J Am Coll Cardiol 1997;30(3):725–32.

[33] Philbin EF. Comprehensive multidisciplinary programs for the management of patients with congestive heart failure. J Gen Intern Med 1999;14(2):130–5.

[34] USDA. Dietary guidelines for Americans. In: United States Department of Agriculture. 6th edition. Washington, DC: U.S. Government Printing Office; 2005.

[35] Lichtenstein AH, Appel LJ, Brands M, et al. Diet and lifestyle recommendations revision 2006: a scientific statement from the American Heart Association Nutrition Committee. Circulation 2006;114(1):82–96.

[36] Travers B, O'Loughlin C, Murphy NF, et al. Fluid restriction in the management of decompensated heart failure: no impact on time to clinical stability. J Card Fail 2007;13(2):128–32.

[37] Ceconi C, Curello S, Bachetti T, et al. Tumor necrosis factor in congestive heart failure: a mechanism of disease for the new millennium? Prog Cardiovasc Dis 1998;41(1 Suppl 1): 25–30.

[38] Anker SD, Ponikowski P, Varney S, et al. Wasting as independent risk factor for mortality in chronic heart failure. Lancet 1997;349(9058):1050–3.

[39] Mustafa I, Leverve X. Metabolic and nutritional disorders in cardiac cachexia. Nutrition 2001;17(9):756–60.

[40] Basu A, Devaraj S, Jialal I. Dietary factors that promote or retard inflammation. Arterioscler Thromb Vasc Biol 2006;26(5):995–1001.

[41] Giugliano D, Ceriello A, Esposito K. The effects of diet on inflammation: emphasis on the metabolic syndrome. J Am Coll Cardiol 2006;48(4):677–85.

[42] Simopoulos AP. The importance of the ratio of omega-6/omega-3 essential fatty acids. Biomed Pharmacother 2002;56(8):365–79.
[43] Calder PC. Immunoregulatory and anti-inflammatory effects of n-3 polyunsaturated fatty acids. Braz J Med Biol Res 1998;31:467–90.
[44] Heller AR, Theilen HJ, Koch T. Fish or chips? News Physiol Sci 2003;18(2):50–4.
[45] Freeman LM, Rush JE, Kehayias JJ, et al. Nutritional alterations and the effect of fish oil supplementation in dogs with heart failure. J Vet Intern Med 1998;12(6):440–8.
[46] Mehra MR, Lavie CJ, Ventura HO, et al. Fish oils produce anti-inflammatory effects and improve body weight in severe heart failure. J Heart Lung Transplant 2006;25(7):834–8.
[47] Lennie TA, Chung ML, Habash DL, et al. Dietary fat intake and proinflammatory cytokine levels in patients with heart failure. J Card Fail 2005;11(8):613–8.
[48] Pischon T, Hankinson SE, Hotamisligil GS, et al. Habitual dietary intake of n-3 and n-6 fatty acids in relation to inflammatory markers among US men and women. Circulation 2003;108:155–60.
[49] Han SN, Leka LS, Lichtenstein AH, et al. Effect of hydrogenated and saturated, relative to polyunsaturated, fat on immune and inflammatory responses of adults with moderate hyper-cholesterolemia. J Lipid Res 2002;43(3):445–52.
[50] Baer DJ, Judd JT, Clevidence BA, et al. Dietary fatty acids affect plasma markers of inflammation in healthy men fed controlled diets: a randomized crossover study. Am J Clin Nutr 2004;79(6):969–73.
[51] Kris-Etherton PM, Harris WS, Appel LJ. Fish consumption, fish oil, omega-3 fatty acids, and cardiovascular disease. Circulation 2002;106(21):2747–57.
[52] Supreme Scientific Health Council MoHaWoG. Dietary guidelines for adults in Greece. Available at: http://www.nut.uoa.gr/english/GreekGuid.htm. Accessed June 21, 2007.
[53] Chrysohoou C, Panagiotakos DB, Pitsavos C, et al. Adherence to the Mediterranean diet attenuates inflammation and coagulation process in healthy adults: The ATTICA Study. J Am Coll Cardiol 2004;44(1):152–8.
[54] Esposito K, Marfella R, Ciotola M, et al. Effect of a Mediterranean-style diet on endothelial dysfunction and markers of vascular inflammation in the metabolic syndrome: a randomized trial. JAMA 2004;292:1440–6.
[55] McNurlan MA, Garlick PJ. Protein synthesis and degradation. In: Stipanuk MH, editor. Biochemical and physiological aspects of human nutrition. 1st edition. Philadelphia: WB Saunders; 2000. p. 211–32.
[56] May PE, Barber A, D'Olimpio JT, et al. Reversal of cancer-related wasting using oral supplementation with a combination of beta-hydroxy-beta-methylbutyrate, arginine, and glutamine. Am J Surg 2002;183(4):471–9.
[57] Clark RH, Feleke G, Din M, et al. Nutritional treatment for acquired immunodeficiency virus-associated wasting using beta-hydroxy beta-methylbutyrate, glutamine, and arginine: a randomized, double-blind, placebo-controlled study. JPEN J Parenter Enteral Nutr 2000;24(3):133–9.
[58] Laviano A, Muscaritoli M, Cascino A, et al. Branched-chain amino acids: the best compromise to achieve anabolism? Curr Opin Clin Nutr Metab Care 2005;8(4):408–14.
[59] Institute of Medicine. Protein and amino acids. dietary reference intakes for energy, carbohydrate, fiber, fat, protein, amino acids (macronutrients). Washington, DC: National Academies Press; 2005. p. 589–768.
[60] Aquilani R, Opasich C, Verri M, et al. Is nutritional intake adequate in chronic heart failure patients? J Am Coll Cardiol 2003;42(7):1218–23.
[61] Gorelik O, Almoznino-Sarafian D, Feder I, et al. Dietary intake of various nutrients in older patients with congestive heart failure. Cardiology 2003;99(4):177–81.
[62] Mitchell MK. Aging and older adults. In: Alexopoulos Y, editor. Nutrition across the lifespan. 2nd edition. Philadelphia: WB Saunders; 2003. p. 429–70.
[63] Witte KK, Nikitin NP, Parker AC, et al. The effect of micronutrient supplementation on quality-of-life and left ventricular function in elderly patients with chronic heart failure. Eur Heart J 2005;26(21):2238–44.

[64] Costello RB, Moser-Veillon PB, DiBianco R. Magnesium supplementation in patients with congestive heart failure. J Am Coll Nutr 1997;16(1):22–31.

[65] Witte KK, Clark AL. Micronutrients and their supplementation in chronic cardiac failure. An update beyond theoretical perspectives. Heart Fail Rev 2006;11(1):65–74.

[66] Lennie TA, Moser DK, Habash DL, et al. Nutritional adequacy of low sodium diets in patients with heart failure. Circulation 2003;108(Suppl):IV-503.

[67] Institute of Medicine. Vitamin D. Dietary reference intakes for calcium, phosphorus, magnesium, vitamin D and fluoride. Washington DC: National Academy Press; 1997. p. 250–287.

[68] Zittermann A, Schleithoff SS, Koerfer R. Vitamin D insufficiency in congestive heart failure: why and what to do about it? Heart Fail Rev 2006;11(1):25–33.

[69] Zittermann A, Schleithoff SS, Tenderich G, et al. Low vitamin D status: a contributing factor in the pathogenesis of congestive heart failure? J Am Coll Cardiol 2003;41(1):105–12.

[70] Park C, Oh Y, Shin Y, et al. Intravenous calcitriol regresses myocardial hypertrophy in hemodialysis patients with secondary hyperparathyroidism. Am J Kidney Dis 1999;33(1): 73–81.

[71] Schleithoff SS, Zittermann A, Tenderich G, et al. Vitamin D supplementation improves cytokine profiles in patients with congestive heart failure: a double-blind, randomized, placebo-controlled trial. Am J Clin Nutr 2006;83(4):754–9.

[72] Stio M, Martinesi M, Bruni S, et al. Interaction among vitamin D3 analogue KH 1060, TNF-[alpha], and vitamin D receptor protein in peripheral blood mononuclear cells of inflammatory bowel disease patients. Int Immunopharmacol 2006;6(7):1083–92.

[73] Zhu Y, Mahon BD, Froicu M, et al. Calcium and 1 alpha,25-dihydroxyvitamin D3 target the TNF-alpha pathway to suppress experimental inflammatory bowel disease. Eur J Immunol 2005;35:217–24.

[74] Lefebvre d'Hellencourt C, Montero-Menei CN, Bernard R, et al. Vitamin D3 inhibits proinflammatory cytokines and nitric oxide production by the EOC13 microglial cell line. J Neurosci Res 2003;71(4):575–82.

[75] Takahashi K, Horiuchi H, Ohta T, et al. 1α,25-dihydroxyvitamin D3 suppresses interleukin-1β-induced interleukin-8 in human whole blood: an involvement of erythrocytes in the inhibition. Immunopharmacol Immunotoxicol 2002;24(1):1–15.

[76] de Lorgeril M, Salen P. Selenium and antioxidant defenses as major mediators in the development of chronic heart failure. Heart Fail Rev 2006;11(1):13–7.

[77] Keith ME, Jeejeebhoy KN, Langer A, et al. A controlled clinical trial of vitamin E supplementation in patients with congestive heart failure. Am J Clin Nutr 2001;73(2):219–24.

[78] Lonn E, Bosch J, Yusuf S, et al. Effects of long-term vitamin E supplementation on cardiovascular events and cancer: a randomized controlled trial. JAMA 2005;293(11): 1338–47.

[79] Miller ER, Pastor-Barriuso R, Dalal D, et al. Meta-analysis: high-dosage vitamin E supplementation may increase all-cause mortality. Ann Intern Med 2005;142(1):37–46.

[80] Hayden KM, Welsh-Bohmer KA, Wengreen HJ, et al. Risk of mortality with vitamin E supplements: the Cache County study. Am J Med 2007;120(2):180–4.

[81] Seligmann H, Halkin H, Rauchfleisch S, et al. Thiamine deficiency in patients with congestive heart failure receiving long-term furosemide therapy: a pilot study. Am J Med 1991; 91(2):151–5.

[82] Allard ML, Jeejeebhoy KN, Sole MJ. The management of conditioned nutritional requirements in heart failure. Heart Fail Rev 2006;11(1):75–82.

[83] Gibelin P, Serre S, Candito M, et al. Prognostic value of homocysteinemia in patients with congestive heart failure. Clin Chem Lab Med 2006;44(7):813–6.

[84] Herrmann M, Muller S, Kindermann I, et al. Plasma B vitamins and their relation to the severity of chronic heart failure. Am J Clin Nutr 2007;85(1):117–23.

[85] Nilsson-Ehle H. Age-related changes in cobalamin (vitamin B12) handling. Implications for therapy. Drugs Aging 1998;12(4):277–92.

[86] Kenchaiah S, Evans JC, Levy D, et al. Obesity and the risk of heart failure. N Engl J Med 2002;347(5):305–13.

[87] Alpert MA, Terry BE, Mulekar M, et al. Cardiac morphology and left ventricular function in normotensive morbidly obese patients with and without congestive heart failure, and effect of weight loss. Am J Cardiol 1997;80(6):736–40.

[88] Zee KJV, Kohno T, Fischer E, et al. Tumor necrosis factor soluble receptors circulate during experimental and clinical inflammation and can protect against excessive tumor necrosis factor-alpha in vitro and in vivo. Proc Natl Acad Sci U S A 1992;89(11):4845–9.

[89] Opal SM, DePalo VA. Anti-inflammatory cytokines. Chest 2000;117(4):1162–72.

[90] Lennie TA. Nutritional recommendations for patients with heart failure. J Cardiovasc Nurs 2006;21(4):261–8.

[91] Habbu A, Lakkis NM, Dokainish H. The obesity paradox: fact or fiction? Am J Cardiol 2006;98(7):944–8.

[92] Lavie CJ, Mehra MR, Milani RV. Obesity and heart failure prognosis: paradox or reverse epidemiology? Eur Heart J 2005;26(1):5–7.

[93] Krumholz HM, Chen YT, Wang Y, et al. Predictors of readmission among elderly survivors of admission with heart failure. Am Heart J 2000;139(1 Pt 1):72–7.

[94] Shindler DM, Kostis JB, Yusuf S, et al. Diabetes mellitus, a predictor of morbidity and mortality in the Studies of Left Ventricular Dysfunction (SOLVD) Trials and Registry. Am J Cardiol 1996;77(11):1017–20.

NURSING
CLINICS
OF NORTH AMERICA

ELSEVIER
SAUNDERS

Nurs Clin N Am 43 (2008) 133–153

Medication Adherence in Patients Who Have Heart Failure: a Review of the Literature

Jia-Rong Wu, PhD, RN[a,b,*],
Debra K. Moser, DNSc, RN, FAAN[a],
Terry A. Lennie, PhD, RN[a],
Patricia V. Burkhart, PhD, RN[a]

[a]College of Nursing, University of Kentucky, 527 CON Building,
760 Rose Street, Lexington, KY 40536-0232, USA
[b]Department of Nursing, Chung Jung Christian University, Tainan, Taiwan

Heart failure (HF) is a serious health care problem and the most rapidly growing cardiovascular disorder in the United States. More than 5 million Americans have HF, and approximately 550,000 new cases occur each year [1]. In 2007, the estimated direct and indirect cost of HF in the United States was $33.2 billion [1,2]. The incidence of HF approaches 10 out of 1000 people older than age 65 [1,2], and HF is the major hospital discharge diagnosis for older adults. As a consequence, the aging of the population will result in a marked increase in the incidence and prevalence of HF [2,3].

The suggested treatment goals for HF include symptom control, maintenance or improvement of quality of life, reducing morbidity and mortality, and slowing the progressive nature of cardiac remodeling that is a hallmark of this condition [4]. A comprehensive care approach and multiple medications are required to meet these goals. To achieve better outcomes, optimal patient adherence to prescribed medications is vital.

Medication nonadherence, however, is common in patients who have HF [5–7]. Estimated medication nonadherence rates range from 10% to 93%, with most investigators citing rates of about 40% to 60% [8–21]. Available data indicate that nonadherence plays a major role in preventable rehospitalizations [22]. These findings demonstrate the importance of improving

* Corresponding author. College of Nursing, University of Kentucky, 527 CON Building, 760 Rose Street, Lexington, KY 40536-0232.
E-mail address: jwu4@uky.edu (J-R. Wu).

medication adherence in patients who have HF. An important first step to improving medication adherence is determining the factors that affect adherence. Accordingly, the purposes of this article are to: (1) describe medication nonadherence rates among patients who have HF, (2) critically review the literature on factors affecting medication adherence in patients who have HF, and (3) depict limitations of existing literature.

Method

The Medline (1966–2007), Cumulative Index to Nursing and Allied Health (CINAHL) (1982–2007), and PsycInfo (1872–2007) databases were searched, using the terms "heart failure," "medication adherence," and "medication compliance." The major focus of this review was articles in which variables associated with medication adherence/compliance in patients who had heart failure were investigated. Qualitative or quantitative research articles dealing directly with medication adherence or medication compliance in HF were chosen. Because the relationships between medication adherence and health care provider, patient relationships, and patient depression and anxiety were rarely studied in patients who had HF, research articles published on these subjects in patients who had cardiac disease in general were included in this review. This literature review is organized according to a framework of medication adherence (ie, a five-dimension adherence model) based on the report of the World Health Organization (WHO) on adherence to long-term therapies [23]. The five dimensions of this framework are: (1) socioeconomic factors, (2) health care system-related factors, (3) condition-related factors, (4) treatment-related factors, and (5) patient-related factors (Fig. 1).

The abstracts of 166 articles written in English and having adult subjects were reviewed for relevance. Only research articles were included in this review. Some articles were added by reviewing references of the selected literature. A total of 50 articles were deemed relevant and were included in the review.

Definition of medication adherence

A commonly used definition of medication compliance is the extent to which the patient's medication-taking behavior coincides with the prescribed medication regimen [23–25]. This definition is not patient-centered and emphasizes the paternalistic role of health care providers. Therefore, recent literature suggests using the term "adherence" instead of compliance. Medication adherence is defined as the extent to which the patient's medication-taking behavior corresponds with an agreed medication regimen from a health care provider [23,24]. The main difference between adherence and compliance is that adherence requires the patient's agreement to the prescribed medication regimen [23]. Medication adherence is patient's active

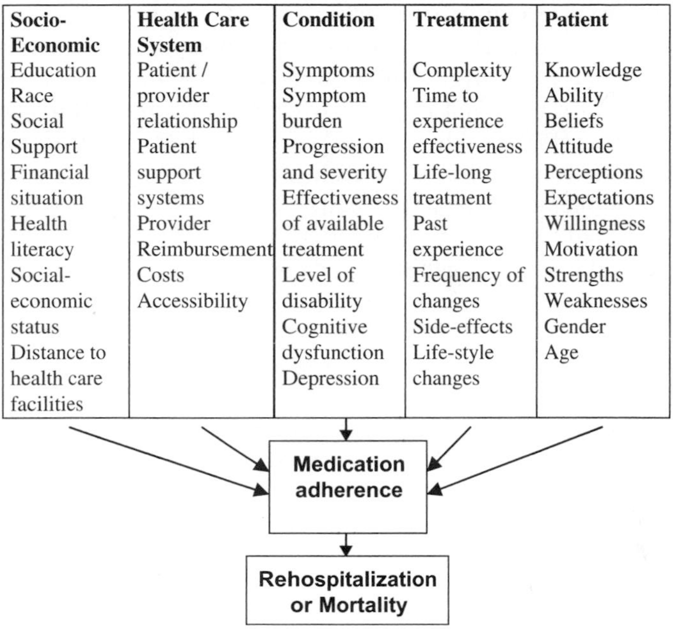

Socio-Economic	Health Care System	Condition	Treatment	Patient
Education	Patient /	Symptoms	Complexity	Knowledge
Race	provider	Symptom	Time to	Ability
Social	relationship	burden	experience	Beliefs
Support	Patient	Progression	effectiveness	Attitude
Financial	support	and severity	Life-long	Perceptions
situation	systems	Effectiveness	treatment	Expectations
Health	Provider	of available	Past	Willingness
literacy	Reimbursement	treatment	experience	Motivation
Social-	Costs	Level of	Frequency of	Strengths
economic	Accessibility	disability	changes	Weaknesses
status		Cognitive	Side-effects	Gender
Distance to		dysfunction	Life-style	Age
health care		Depression	changes	
facilities				

```
                    Medication
                    adherence

                Rehospitalization
                   or Mortality
```

Fig. 1. WHO's multidimensional adherence model and rehospitalization.

choice in taking prescribed medications [23,24]. There are many different medication-taking behaviors that can be considered nonadherent. Nonadherence includes dosage errors (underuse and overuse), not having a prescription filled, interruption of treatment, failure to take medications at specified times, taking medication at incorrect intervals [26], and taking medications not prescribed. In this review, any deviation from the prescribed medication regimen was considered medication nonadherence.

Medication nonadherence rates

It is difficult to come to a valid conclusion about medication adherence rates in patients who have HF because of methodological weaknesses in the research. Researchers have used different operational definitions of medication adherence, and some failed to include any operational definition of medication adherence in their studies [27–30]. Medication adherence has been measured using self-report and a variety of more objective measures, resulting in widely varying reports of medication adherence rates.

Using self-report measures, medication nonadherence rates were reported to be anywhere from 4% to 54% in 13 studies [9,10,12,13,21,31–38]. A variety of different questionnaires were used to measure self-reported adherence. Investigators did not report raw adherence rates; rather, the percentage who were adherent verse not adherent was based on an arbitrary cutoff point, and this cutoff point differed by study.

Pharmacy refill is an objective measure of adherence. Pharmacy refill data are extracted from patients' records from pharmacy claims database. There are two ways to use pharmacy refill history to represent patients' medication adherence. The first method is pharmacy refill rate, also called medication possession ratio (MPR). The number of days when medication (filled at the pharmacies over the period of study time) was available to patients is taken as the numerator. The denominator is the total length of time patients are in the study [27,39]. The second method is cumulative mean gap ratio [40]. The cumulative mean gap ratio for a specified time period is calculated by dividing the number of days that medication is unavailable for consumption (because of a delayed refill) by the total number of days during the time period [40]. Using the pharmacy refill measure, medication nonadherence rates have been reported to range from 2% to 90% in eight studies [14,19,27,29,30,41–43]. Pharmacy refill adherence was analyzed as a continuous or a dichotomous variable. The cutoff point for adherence or nonadherence was inconsistently defined and ranged from 75% to 90%. Moreover, investigators used different methods to calculate refill adherence rate, such as cumulative medication acquisition or cumulative multiple-refill interval gap, making it difficult to compare results.

The medication event monitoring system (MEMS) is a novel approach to assessing adherence [44]. The system includes a special container with a microprocessor that records each time that the cap is removed from a medication bottle [45,46]. Using the MEMS, medication nonadherence rates range from 2% to 60% in four studies [17,47–49]. All studies treated medication adherence rate as a continuous variable, although some investigators reported mean adherence [17,47–49], and some reported median adherence [49]. The MEMS can give a full picture of a patient's medication adherence by providing data such the percentage of prescribed doses taken, the percentage of days the correct number of doses is taken, and the percentage of doses taken at the correct time. Not all of the researchers reported these data, however. Thus, a full picture of a patient's medication taking behavior was not seen. Also, making comparisons between studies using the MEMS measure is impossible.

Pill count is another objective and commonly used method for evaluating medication adherence. Using pill count, patients are asked to return medications to the study center or a home visit is arranged so that the pills left in the medication bottle can be counted and compare with the prescription and the date patients refill medication. Using pill count measure, medication nonadherence rates ranged from 15% to 73% [8,18].

In summary, medication nonadherence rates in patients who have HF vary dramatically from 2% to 90%, depending on how adherence is measured and defined. The desired level of medication adherence remains unknown, however. Without this information, it is difficult for researchers and clinicians to set a goal to improve medication adherence. It is necessary for future investigators to determine the level of medication adherence required to achieve optimal outcomes in patients who have HF.

Factors influencing medication adherence

Despite the number of prior interventions aimed at improving medication adherence, adherence rates remain low. A major reason for this could be that investigators have not systematically examined factors affecting adherence using an appropriate theory and multivariate approach. A five-dimension adherence model from the WHO report on adherence to long-term therapies [23] was used to guide this study. Although there are multiple health behavior models, there is no other published model specific to medication adherence in HF. In one review article, Leventhal and colleagues [50] categorized factors influencing medication adherence based on the WHO model from a review of HF literature (see Fig. 1). The five dimensions of the multidimensional adherence model (MAM) are: (1) socioeconomic factors, (2) health care system-related factors, (3) condition-related factors, (4) treatment-related factors, and (5) patient-related factors. There are multiple indicators in each dimension. The literature review reported here was organized based on the categories delineated in the MAM (Table 1).

Socioeconomic factors

The MAM includes multiple indicators under the category of socioeconomic factors (see Fig. 1). Only household income, marital status, living alone, social support, education, and race were investigated as potential predictors of adherence in patients who had HF [8–10,18,21,30,35,37,48,49,51,52,55].

Household income

Few investigators have examined the relationship between income and medication adherence, and the results are inconsistent [10,35,48]. In one study of 169 patients [48], the relationship was tested in a multivariate model and medication adherence was measured objectively using a MEMS. The investigators found that as household income increased, adherence increased. Contrary findings were reported in two other studies in which the relationship was tested in a multivariate model (N = 209) [35] and in a bivariate model (N = 401) [10]. Although the large sample sizes are strengths of each study, medication adherence was measured subjectively by self-report in both, a method of medication adherence that is open to critique because it often results in overestimation of adherence. Income did not predict adherence in either study [10,35].

Marital status

Only one group of investigators studied the relationship between marital status and adherence; a bivariate model and self-report measure was used in a large sample (N = 401) of HF patients [10]. Being married was associated with greater adherence. In a meta-analysis of the impact of marital status on adherence in a variety of patient groups, being married was associated with greater adherence [73]. These results might be explained by the fact that

Table 1
Factors influencing medication adherence

Variables	Findings
Socioeconomic factors:	
Household income	No consistent result [10,35,48]
Marital status	Married patients were more adherent [10].
Living status	Patients who live with someone were more adherent [8–10].
Social support	More social support, more adherent [9,30,37,51,52]
Education	More education, more adherent [10,21,35,49]
Race	No consistent result [8,18,21,48]
Health care system-related factors:	
Patient-provider interaction	No relationship between patient-provider interaction and medication adherence [53]
Patient satisfaction	Higher patient satisfaction with health care received, more adherent [54]
Trust in health care providers	Higher trust in health care providers, more adherent [52,55]
Patient-provider communication	No consistent results [30,52,55,56]
Condition-related factors:	
Symptom severity	More severity of symptoms, more adherent [14,35,57,58]
Comorbidity	No consistent result [14,35,43]
Depression	More depressed, less adherent [59–64]
Anxiety	No association between anxiety and medication adherence [65]
Treatment-related factors:	
Perceived effects or side effects	Perceived more benefits and fewer side effects, more adherent [13,30–32,52,64,66–68]
Previous hospitalization	With previous hospitalization, more adherent [14,19]
Complexity	
Pills taken per day	Higher number of pills taken, less adherent [18,67,68]
Multiple medications	No consistent result [9,19,43]
Medication frequency	No consistent result [17,48,69,70]
Packaging	Medication adherence was better with unit-of-use packaging [28,67,69]
Medication container	Difficulty removing the tops from medication containers was a major reason for nonadherence [13,67].
Cost of medication	Higher medication cost, less adherent [9,30,32,37,42,52,57,66,71]
Patient-related factors:	
Age	No consistent result [10,12,14,18,19,21,32,35,67]
Gender	No consistent result [10,12,19,21,35,43]
Forgetfulness	One of the most common barriers to adherence [9,31,32,37,52,67,68]
Knowledge	No consistent result [10,12,13,31,37,52,68,72]
Motivation for well-being	Higher motivation for increasing well-being, better medication adherence [51,58,68]
Routine	Not fit in patients' routine, more likely to be nonadherent [31,52,68,70]

married patients had their spouses to help them, remind them, emotionally support them, and provide motivation to remain healthy.

Living alone

In a comprehensive meta-analysis involving hundreds of patients who had a variety of diagnoses, living alone was associated with a risk of nonadherence to medication [73]. The odds of adherence for those living with another person were 1.38 times higher compared with those living alone. This finding has been confirmed by most investigators who have specifically examined the relationship in HF [8–10]. In each of these studies sample sizes greater than 120 were used. In contrast, one group of investigators found that adherence decreased as the number of persons living in the household increased, and that living alone was associated with the highest adherence rates [48]. In this study, the relationship was tested in a multivariate model, and medication adherence was measured by MEMS, but the number of HF patients living alone in this sample was only five, seriously limiting the validity of the study's findings. Thus, the preponderance of evidence suggests that living alone is a risk factor for nonadherence.

Social support

In a comprehensive meta-analysis of studies of adherence among various patients who had chronic diseases [73], practical, emotional, and unidimensional social support, as well as family cohesiveness and conflict, marital status, and living arrangements were associated with adherence. Practical social support had the highest correlation with adherence; the odds of adherence were 3.6 times higher among those who received practical support than among those who did not. In studies conducted specifically among patients who had HF, the majority of investigators found that social support was significantly related to medication adherence [9,30,37,51,52]. Lack of social support was one of the most common factors in medication nonadherence [9,30,51].

Education

Education level is related consistently to adherence in that patients with more education were more likely, by self-report, to adhere to their prescribed medication regimens [10,21,35,49].

Race

The relationship between race and medication adherence was examined in four studies [8,18,21,48] and the results were inconsistent. In two studies, white participants were more adherent than minority participants [8,18]. This relationship was tested in a multivariate model using an objective measure of adherence—pill count—in both. In contrast, another group of investigators using the MEMS and multivariate model testing reported that black participants were more adherent [48]. A fourth group found that race was not related to medication adherence [21]. Based on the available literature, it is difficult to draw a conclusion about the relationship between race and adherence.

In summary, the strongest sets of socioeconomic factors related to adherence are social support and related constructs (ie, living alone or not and marital status). Presence of adequate social support, living with others, and being married are all associated with better adherence. Higher education level is also associated with better adherence. The findings regarding the relationship of race and income to adherence are inconsistent. The relationships between medication adherence and other important factors (eg, health literacy, distance to health care facilities) in the socioeconomic category were not discussed in the literature.

Health care system-related factors

The patient-provider relationship has been acknowledged by most investigators as an important factor in medication adherence. The dimensions of the patient-provider relationship included in this review are patient-provider interaction, patient satisfaction, trust in health care providers, and patient-provider communication. HF patients, however, have rarely been studied. There are three research studies published on this subject in patients who had cardiac disease in general [53–55] and three in HF specifically [30,52,56]. Because of the lack of HF specific literature in this area, all six articles are reviewed here.

Patient-provider interaction

The impact of a positive patient-provider interaction on medication adherence has been reported in only one study [53]. Patients remembered physicians' directions better when the physician was more friendly and allowed them to act as partners during interviews. Ultimately, however, there was no relationship between this aspect of patient-provider interaction and patients' medication adherence [53].

Patient satisfaction

Patient satisfaction with health care in general has been found to be a significant predictor of medication adherence measured by self-report, provider-report, and pharmacy refill [54]. Patient satisfaction with the health care they received and belief that providers were qualified, competent, and responsive to needs were related to better medication adherence.

Trust in health care providers

Although it is commonly assumed that patient-provider trust improves adherence, this assumption has been tested in only two studies in cardiac patients [52,55]. In one qualitative study [52], investigators found that a relationship characterized by trust between the patient and provider was

a motivating factor for maintaining a high level of adherence. The participants also emphasized the need for health care providers to be knowledgeable and answer all questions, as well as to show genuine concern for their
well-being [52]. Other investigators found that patients who took their
medication regularly appeared to have a higher regard for their health
care providers. They believed drugs would not be prescribed unnecessarily
and took their medication because their doctor "told me to take it" [55].

Patient-provider communication
    In two qualitative studies, focus groups have been used to examine pa-
tient-provider communication and self-reported medication adherence
[52,55]. Good patient-provider communication within a trusting relationship was positively associated with medication adherence. Similarly, patients
who experienced communication problems and lacked a meaningful relationship with their health care provider have been reported to be much
less adherent [56]. In Simpson and colleagues' [30] quantitative study, however, the investigators could not find a significant relationship between communication with health care provider and medication adherence because of
the very high level of adherence to drug use. Therefore, these results suggest
that good patient-provider communication appears fundamental to enhancing adherence, but is not sufficient to produce the adherence.
    From the reviewed literature, it is apparent that building a trusting pa-
tient-provider relationship is essential to medication adherence. There is,
however, a need for clearer definitions of the specific aspects of health
care provider-patient interactions that improve adherence.

Condition-related factors

    Symptom severity, comorbidity, depression, and anxiety are commonly
accepted as factors affecting medication adherence, but these have not
been examined systematically.

Symptom severity
    Physical discomfort might be an important internal cue to action. In all
of the studies in which investigators examined the relationship between
symptom severity and medication adherence, symptom severity was consistently related to medication adherence [14,35,57,58], regardless of how
adherence was measured. One illustration of the power of symptoms to
influence behavior was found in a study of drug use behavior under the
constraints of a Medicaid prescription cap [57]. In this study, individuals
decided which medications to take or not based on symptom severity [57].
In another study, investigators examined the relationship between New
York Heart Association (NYHA) functional class and medication adherence, and found that the higher the NYHA functional class, the less the
risk of medication nonadherence [14].

Comorbidity

Inconsistent results have been reported in the studies examining the relationship between comorbidity and medication adherence [14,35,43]. In two studies [14,43], patients who had HF who had hyperlipidemia, asthma/ chronic obstructive pulmonary disease (COPD), or prior myocardial infarction (MI) were more likely to be nonadherent. The relationship was tested in a multivariate model using large samples in both studies (N = 311 and 869, respectively). Medication adherence was measured by pharmacy refill record [43] and self-report [14]. Other researchers, however, have reported that comorbidity was unrelated to medication adherence [35]. In this study, the relationship was tested in a multivariate model using a large sample (N = 209), and medication adherence was measured by self-report questionnaire. The inconsistent results might be caused by differences in the way comorbidities were assessed. In one study, comorbidities were assessed by asking patients what concomitant diseases they had [14]. In a second study, the investigators specifically asked patients whether they had prior MI, atrial fibrillation, diabetes mellitus, renal insufficiency, and hypertension [43]. In the third study, comorbidity was measured using the Charlson Index to categorize participants [35]. Based on these studies, it is difficult to draw a conclusion about the relationship between comorbidity and adherence.

Depression

In a meta-analysis of the relationship between depression or anxiety and adherence in medically ill patients, depression, but not anxiety, was a predictor of nonadherence [59]. An additional six studies not included in that meta-analysis focusing on either HF, heart disease, or high risk for heart disease were found [60–65]. In all but one study [65], depression was related to medication nonadherence. The negative study was conducted among individuals who had familial hypercholesterolemia who did not have overt heart disease [65]. Based on results from studies, depressed patients who have overt heart disease are less adherent to prescribed medications.

Anxiety

Only one study was found examining the effect of anxiety on adherence. Investigators found no association between anxiety and medication adherence in a group of patients who had familial hypercholesterolemia [65]. In this study, the relationship was tested in a bivariate model; medication adherence was measured by self-report scale with a large sample (N = 336).

To date, symptom severity and depression are the only condition-related factors that have been consistently demonstrated to be associated with adherence. Less symptomatic patients and those who are depressed are more likely to be nonadherent.

Treatment-related factors

The relationships between medication adherence and treatment-related factors such as the perceived beneficial effects or side effects of medication, previous hospitalization, and characteristics of medication (ie, number of pills taken per day, multiple medications, frequency of dosing, packaging, medication container, and cost of medication) were examined by a number of investigators.

Perceived effects or side effects of medication

A number of investigators have examined the relationship between perceived beneficial effects or side effects of medication with medication adherence [13,30–32,52,64,66–68]. In each of these studies, investigators noted that patients who experienced side effects were less adherent. Patients skipped or delayed taking their medications when they experienced side effects [68]. Other patients lost confidence in new prescriptions when their condition failed to improve dramatically [52]. When patients perceived that medications were ineffective, they stopped taking them [13,31,52]. Thus, it is clear that patients who perceived greater benefit and fewer side effects were more adherent.

Previous hospitalization

In two studies, investigators examined the relationship of previous hospitalization with medication adherence [14,19]. Medication adherence rates were higher in patients with previous hospital or nursing home stays, and the relationships were tested using multivariate models, objective measures of adherence, and large samples (N = 7247, 311, respectively) [14,19].

Characteristics of medication
Number of pills taken per day. As the number of pills taken per day increases, medication adherence decreases [18,67,68]. One reason may be that the complexity of managing multiple medications makes it difficult to follow the medication regimen. For example, in a qualitative study, participants stated that taking too many pills in a day made it difficult to cope with the treatment regimen, thereby reducing adherence [68].

Multiple medications. Studies of the relationship between multiple medication prescriptions and medication adherence have had inconsistent results [9,19,43]. Medication nonadherence rate was significantly higher when patients used two or more medications [9], but other investigators have found that when patients concurrently used other medications like angiotensin-converting enzyme inhibitors, antihyperlipidemic agents, or multiple agents for HF, they were more likely to adhere to their medication regimens [19,43]. Being prescribed multiple medications may alter patients' perceptions so that they believe their condition is more severe, and as a consequence they might be more adherent. A high number of pills taken per day may impede medication adherence, however. Thus, further research is needed to determine the interaction of number of prescriptions, number of pills per day, and patients' perceptions of the implications of these prescribing patterns.

Frequency. Four groups of investigators have studied the relationship between medication frequency and medication adherence [17,48,69,70] with inconsistent findings. In one study, investigators found that two or fewer medication administration times was an independent predictor of nonadherence [70]. To the contrary, other investigators found that as frequency of dosing per day increased, adherence decreased [17,48,69]. Based on results from the majority of the studies in which multivariate analysis was used and objective measure of adherence was employed, it appears that increasing frequency of daily dosing impedes adherence.

Packaging. Investigators have demonstrated that medication adherence suffers when the package, size, and color of tablets differ for the same medication [67]. Medication adherence rates have been found to be better when unit-of-use packaging [69] was used. Investigators have also found that patients preferred once-daily, single-capsule, and fixed-dose medications [28]. Based on the results, even factors that seem trivial, such as medication packaging, may be important to medication adherence.

Medication container. Patients are less adherent when they experience difficulty opening medication containers [13,67]. In one study, 10.1% of the participants could not open at least one medication container [67]. Patients have the most difficulty opening "push and turn" bottles [67], and have reported needing to ask for assistance to get into the bottle [13]. Based on these results, medication adherence might be improved by using easier-to-open medication containers.

Cost of medication. In nine studies, investigators found that high medication cost was one of the most important barriers related to medication adherence [9,30,32,37,42,52,57,66,71]. Some patients report cutting down on food to pay for drugs [52]. As many as 42% in one study did not fill their prescriptions when their medication costs exceeded the limits of the Medicaid prescription cap, slightly fewer changed the way medication was taken (37%), and some took other people's medication (11%) [57].

Other treatment-related factors
Patients who used two or more pharmacies tend to be nonadherent [9]. Likewise, frequent changes in drug prescriptions during hospital stay and after discharge contributed to nonadherence. Patients who had difficulty swallowing pills sometimes didn't take their medications. And finally, poor taste of the medication also contributed to nonadherence [13].

In summary, patients who perceived more benefits and fewer side effects from medication were more adherent, as were those who had previous hospitalizations. The number of pills per day, difficulty removing the tops from medication containers, and medication cost are associated with decreased medication adherence. The impact of being prescribed multiple medications or the frequency of daily medications on medication adherence is less clear.

Patient-related factors

The relationships between medication adherence and patient-related factors such as age, gender, patient's ability, beliefs, attitude, perceptions, expectations, willingness, and motivation were examined by a number of investigators.

Age

In nine studies, investigators examined the relationship between age and medication adherence in patients who had HF [10,12,14,18,19,21,32,35,67]. The results were inconsistent. In two studies, younger patients were more adherent to medication prescription [12,14,18,43], but this relationship was not tested using multivariate models. In the one study in this group [18] in which a multivariate model was tested, age, although significantly related to adherence in a bivariate analysis, was unrelated in a multivariate model that included age, ethnicity, marital status, and number of pills taken per days [18]. In another four studies, older patients were more adherent [10,14,19,21]. In three of these studies [14,19,21], this relationship was tested in a multivariate analysis. In one study [19] a multivariate model was tested, a large (N = 7247) sample size was used, and medication adherence was measured objectively. In the remaining three studies, age was not significantly related to medication adherence [32,35,67].

A major limitation common to all of these studies that may contribute to inconsistencies in findings is variable definitions of age groups. With one exception [21], the studies in this group had large sample sizes of more than 100 participants. Only four studies used objective (pill count and pharmacy refill) measures of adherence [14,18,19,67], whereas the remainder used self-report measures. Based on results from studies in which multivariate analyses were used, sample sizes were large, and objective measures of adherence were employed, it appears that older patients are more adherent.

Gender

As with age, findings about the association of gender and medication adherence were inconsistent [10,12,19,21,35,43]. In two studies, men were more adherent than women [12,43]. In one study, this relationship was tested only in a bivariate model and medication adherence was measured by self-report measurement [12]. In the other study, the relationship was tested in multivariate analysis with a large sample and objective measurement of adherence [43]. In contrast, in two studies women were more adherent than men [10,19].

In one study, the relationship was tested in a multivariate model and used an objective measure of adherence [19]. In the other study, the relationship was only tested in a bivariate model and used a self-report measure [10]. Both studies had large samples. In the remaining two studies gender was not a significant predictor of medication adherence [21,35]. Thus, it is difficult to draw a conclusion about the relationship between gender and adherence.

Forgetfulness

Forgetfulness was associated with nonadherence in all of the studies in which the relationship was examined [9,31,32,67], and was one of the most common barriers to adherence [37]. To improve medication-taking behavior, using reminders such as weekly drug dispensers, drug cups, or setting up a room for medication may enhance medication adherence [37,52,68]. Patients who tend to forget to take their medications were more likely to report that another person prepared medication for them [31].

Knowledge

A number of investigators have tested the hypothesis that medication knowledge was important to medication adherence [10,12,13,31,37,52,72]. In two qualitative studies [68,72], participants reported that medication nonadherence was related to their vague or absent understanding of HF and doubts about how to manage their HF. As a result of uncertainty about their HF, many patients expressed the need to learn more about their condition and the prescribed drugs so that their adherence could improve [52]. In a quantitative study, Huang [10] tested the relationship in a bivariate model by self-report measure and found a significant correlation between knowledge and medication adherence. Another group of investigators reported that lack of knowledge was a barrier to medication adherence by self-report measure of medication adherence [37]. In three other studies, however, knowledge of medication was not significantly related to adherence [12,13,31]. These results suggest that knowledge maybe a prerequisite to adherence, but is not sufficient to produce adherence. Additional factors, such as attitude and cues to action, may also be necessary [12,31].

Motivation for increasing well-being

Investigators have primarily examined the relationship between motivation and medication adherence using qualitative studies [51,58,68]. In one qualitative study, motivation to stay out of the hospital was a major facilitator of adherence [68]. In another, investigators found that the absence of motivation contributed to nonadherence [51]. In quantitative investigation, patients who believed that they might get better or have a good quality of life as a result of taking their medications were more willing to adhere to the prescribed regimen [58]. Based on these studies, motivation to stay out of hospital, to get better, and to have a good quality of life appears important to patients' adherence to medication.

Routine

Investigators reported that when medications did not fit into patients' routine, they were more likely to miss taking them [31,52,68,70]. Qualitative studies revealed that patients might intentionally skip or delay a diuretic dose if they had activities planned, because of fear of frequent urination after taking diuretics [52,68].

In summary, patients who were more forgetful or whose medication schedule interfered with their routine were less likely to adhere to their medications. On the contrary, patients who had believed their well-being could improve with medication were more adherent to medication. The relationships between medication adherence and age, gender, and knowledge were inconsistent.

Discussion

Our understanding of the relationships of age, gender, race, and living status with medication adherence is limited because results from studies have been inconsistent in the available literature. Knowledge of medication did not appear to be related directly to medication adherence. As would be expected, forgetfulness was negatively associated with medication adherence. Patients who believe that there are benefits to taking their medications or who do not experience side effects are more adherent, as are those who have high motivation for improving their well-being. Social support was positively related to medication adherence. A good patient-provider relationship, especially one that was perceived as trusting, enhanced medication adherence.

Limitations of existing literature

There are at least five major problems in the study of medication adherence in HF that need to be addressed to improve the quality of research in this area. Many of the inconsistencies in findings about the relationship of medication adherence to the variables studied are related to one or more of these five problems.

The first issue is related to problems with defining the desired levels of medication adherence. At this stage we do not know what level of medication adherence is necessary for individual drug classes to achieve the optimal benefit. There are too few studies on the relationship of medication adherence and subsequent "control" of the condition. The commonly used cutoff point is 80% adherence, above which adherence is thought to be sufficient. The reason for choosing 80% adherence is unclear, and is not based on empirical data. In fact, in many cases, this level of medication adherence is meaningless, and is not based on pharmacologic evidence linking frequency and dose of medication taking with clinical outcomes [74]. If there were a common, agreed upon, and meaningful level of adherence that all investigators used to define adherence, it is likely that some inconsistencies in this literature could be resolved. Further research is needed to determine the level of medication adherence required to achieve optimal outcomes in patients who have HF.

The second issue is related to the measurement of medication adherence. A wide variety of instruments are used to measure medication adherence. Lack of consistency in measurement is a major problem in interpreting results about the impact of various factors on adherence. No ideal measure exists for measuring medication adherence. The most frequently used methods include patient's self-report, pill count, pharmacy refills, drug assays of blood or urine or saliva, and microelectronic monitoring devices in the caps of medication containers [25]. Each of these methods has advantages and disadvantages. Currently, electronic monitoring is the most accurate measure of the patients' chronic medication administration [44]; however, findings based on use of the MEMS cap are confounded by patients' need to remember a secondary activity (opening MEMS caps) in conjunction with the primary activity (taking a pill), and by the possibility that adherence will be artificially inflated when a participant is aware that his or her behavior is being monitored. Thus, either existing instruments need to be refined or a new instrument needs to be developed that adequately measures medication adherence.

The third issue is related to research design. Most studies were cross-sectional in nature. Medication adherence is a dynamic process that is likely to change over time. It is unwise to assume that adherence and factors influencing adherence are stable. Future studies need to be conducted using longitudinal designs.

The fourth issue is related to sample size. Many study results were based on small, homogeneous samples [13,21,37,69]. Generalizability is limited under these circumstances.

The final issue is related to failure of many investigators to consider the complexity of medication adherence. Few investigators examined the interrelationships among the variables that likely influence medication adherence. Instead, investigators have concentrated on examination of the direct, bivariate relationships between medication adherence and individual variables. This approach, although informative for establishing preliminary hypotheses, ultimately results in oversimplification and even misrepresentation of the phenomenon of medication adherence. A more comprehensive approach is warranted to fully understand the determinants associated with medication adherence.

Summary

HF is an important health problem in many countries. The review of the literature on medication adherence in patients who have HF suggests that patients are often nonadherent to medications because of a wide range of factors (see Table 1). Several factors such as age, gender, race, and comorbidity of the patient cannot be changed, but patients who have certain of these characteristics can be considered at high risk for poor medication adherence. Other factors presented in this article can be modified with appropriately designed interventions.

In the category of socioeconomic factors, investigators consistently found that patients who cannot afford medication costs are less likely to adhere to their prescribed medications. Patients who are less educated or have no spouse are more likely to be nonadherent, whereas those with more social support are more adherent. Health care providers can act as supporters to patients, but possibly more important naturally existing social support systems must be enhanced. Family members and other informal caregivers need education about how to promote adherence in the patient. Health care reform may be needed to make medications easier for more patients to buy. Even with Medicare (and its recent prescription reforms) or Medicaid, many elderly patients are unable to afford their daily medications. Many patients are un- or under-insured and face serious crises when diagnosed with a chronic cardiac illness that requires multiple expensive medications.

Within the category of health care system-related factors, the patient-provider relationship is important to medication adherence. Therefore, health care providers need to consider the strong role that developing a trusting relationship with their patients can play in improving medication adherence. Both patient and health care provider must communicate well to build a trusting partnership [75]. This area may be one of the easiest to improve, but requires a concerted effort by health care providers and health care systems to enhance to enhance the quality of provider patient interaction.

For condition-related and treatment-related factors, health care providers can play an important role in making a connection between factors within these two dimensions. For example, health care providers can give patients a thorough and clear explanation about their illnesses and the reasons for medication, and regularly check patients' understanding of what they have been told about treatment. Likewise, providers should give patients the opportunity to raise their concerns and respond to them in a timely, consistent manner. Providers should ask patients about side effects or adverse drug reactions and make changes as needed, while emphasizing the importance of adhering to the revised plan at each follow-up. Also, providers and health care organizations need to advocate for easier opening medication packaging and consistency in packaging.

In the patient-related factor category, patient forgetfulness and conflicts between the requirements of the medication routine and the needs of the patient to meet social demands contribute to nonadherence. Thus, health care providers need to assist patients in determining how to adapt their medication schedule to their social needs, and also need to work to make the medication regimen as uncomplicated as possible. Providers can teach patients about the many medication aids available to improve memory for medication taking.

Medication adherence is a complex behavior. Patients are also complex. What level of adherence to medication optimizes outcomes in patients who have HF remains unknown. It is unreasonable to expect that any one will fully adhere to a recommended medical regimen forever without substantial support, assistance, and information from health care providers and informal caregivers. Most importantly, the treatment regimen must take into consideration patients' expectations for their health, their environment, their understanding of the HF progression, and their ability to follow the prescribed regimen.

References

[1] Rosamond W, Flegal K, Friday G, et al. Heart disease and stroke statistics—2007 update: a report from the American Heart Association Statistics Committee and Stroke Statistics Subcommittee. Circulation 2007;115(5):E69–171.

[2] American Heart Association. Heart disease and stroke statistics—2005 update. Dallas (TX): American Heart Association; 2005.

[3] Remme WJ, McMurray JJ, Rauch B, et al. Public awareness of heart failure in Europe: first results from SHAPE. Eur Heart J 2005;26(22):2413–21.

[4] Stanley M, Prasun M. Heart failure in older adults: keys to successful management. AACN Clin Issues 2002;13(1):94–102.

[5] Chin MH, Goldman L. Factors contributing to the hospitalization of patients with congestive heart failure. Am J Public Health 1997;87(4):643–8.

[6] Cole JA, Norman H, Weatherby LB, et al. Drug copayment and adherence in chronic heart failure: effect on cost and outcomes. Pharmacotherapy 2006;26(8):1157–64.

[7] Li H, Morrow-Howell N, Proctor EK. Post-acute home care and hospital readmission of elderly patients with congestive heart failure. Health Soc Work 2004;29(4):275–85.

[8] Rich MW, Gray DB, Beckham V, et al. Effect of a multidisciplinary intervention on medication compliance in elderly patients with congestive heart failure. Am J Med 1996;101(3):270–6.

[9] Col N, Fanale JE, Kronholm P. The role of medication noncompliance and adverse drug reactions in hospitalizations of the elderly. Arch Intern Med 1990;150(4):841–5.

[10] Huang LH. Medication-taking behavior of the elderly. Kaohsiung J Med Sci 1996;12(7):423–33.

[11] Cline CM, Bjorck-Linne AK, Israelsson BY, et al. Non-compliance and knowledge of prescribed medication in elderly patients with heart failure. Eur J Heart Fail 1999;1(2):145–9.

[12] Gonzalez B, Lupon J, Parajon T, et al. Nurse evaluation of patients in a new multidisciplinary heart failure unit in Spain. Eur J Cardiovasc Nurs 2004;3(1):61–9.

[13] Blenkiron P. The elderly and their medication: understanding and compliance in a family practice. Postgrad Med J 1996;72(853):671–6.

[14] Rodgers PT, Ruffin DM. Medication nonadherence: part II—a pilot study in patients with congestive heart failure. Manag Care Interface 1998;11(9):67–9, 75.

[15] Bonner CJ, Carr B. Medication compliance problems in general practice: detection and intervention by pharmacists and doctors. Aust J Rural Health 2002;10(1):33–8.

[16] Bhagat K, Mazayi-Mupanemunda M. Compliance with medication in patients with heart failure in Zimbabwe. East Afr Med J 2001;78(1):45–8.

[17] Bohachick P, Burke LE, Sereika S, et al. Adherence to angiotensin-converting enzyme inhibitor therapy for heart failure. Prog Cardiovasc Nurs 2002;17(4):160–6.

[18] Graveley EA, Oseasohn CS. Multiple drug regimens: medication compliance among veterans 65 years and older. Res Nurs Health 1991;14(1):51–8.

[19] Monane M, Bohn RL, Gurwitz JH, et al. Noncompliance with congestive heart failure therapy in the elderly. Arch Intern Med 1994;154(4):433–7.

[20] Artinian NT, Harden JK, Kronenberg MW, et al. Pilot study of a web-based compliance monitoring device for patients with congestive heart failure. Heart Lung 2003;32(4):226–33.
[21] Evangelista LS, Berg J, Dracup K. Relationship between psychosocial variables and compliance in patients with heart failure. Heart Lung 2001;30(4):294–301.
[22] Rich MW, Beckham V, Wittenberg C, et al. A multidisciplinary intervention to prevent the re-admission of elderly patients with congestive heart failure. N Engl J Med 1995;333(18):1190–5.
[23] Sabate E. Adherence to long-term therapies: evidence for action. Geneva (Switzerland): World Health Organization; 2003. p. 1–194.
[24] Evangelista LS, Dracup K. A closer look at compliance research in heart failure patients in the last decade. Prog Cardiovasc Nurs 2000;15(3):97–103.
[25] Haynes RB, McDonald HP, Garg AX. Helping patients follow prescribed treatment: clinical applications. JAMA 2002;288(22):2880–3.
[26] Miller NH. Compliance with treatment regimens in chronic asymptomatic diseases. Am J Med 1997;102(2A):43–9.
[27] Struthers AD, Anderson G, MacFadyen RJ, et al. Nonadherence with ACE inhibitor treatment is common in heart failure and can be detected by routine serum ACE activity assays. Heart 1999;82(5):584–8.
[28] Taylor AA, Shoheiber O. Adherence to antihypertensive therapy with fixed-dose amlodipine besylate/benazepril HCl versus comparable component-based therapy. Congest Heart Fail 2003;9(6):324–32.
[29] Butler J, Arbogast PG, Daugherty J, et al. Outpatient utilization of angiotensin-converting enzyme inhibitors among heart failure patients after hospital discharge. J Am Coll Cardiol 2004;43(11):2036–43.
[30] Simpson SH, Johnson JA, Farris KB, et al. Development and validation of a survey to assess barriers to drug use in patients with chronic heart failure. Pharmacotherapy 2002;22(9): 1163–72.
[31] Conn V, Taylor S, Miller R. Cognitive impairment and medication adherence. J Gerontol Nurs 1994;20(7):41–7.
[32] Evangelista L, Doering LV, Dracup K, et al. Compliance behaviors of elderly patients with advanced heart failure. J Cardiovasc Nurs 2003;18(3):197–206, quiz 7–8.
[33] Laramee AS, Levinsky SK, Sargent J, et al. Case management in a heterogeneous congestive heart failure population: a randomized controlled trial. Arch Intern Med 2003;163(7): 809–17.
[34] Ni H, Nauman D, Burgess D, et al. Factors influencing knowledge of and adherence to self-care among patients with heart failure. Arch Intern Med 1999;159(14):1613–9.
[35] Rockwell JM, Riegel B. Predictors of self-care in persons with heart failure. Heart Lung 2001;30(1):18–25.
[36] Svarstad BL, Chewning BA, Sleath BL, et al. The brief medication questionnaire: a tool for screening patient adherence and barriers to adherence. Patient Educ Couns 1999;37(2): 113–24.
[37] Welsh JD, Heiser RM, Schooler MP, et al. Characteristics and treatment of patients with heart failure in the emergency department. J Emerg Nurs 2002;28(2):126–31.
[38] Hulka BS, Cassel JC, Kupper LL, et al. Communication, compliance, and concordance between physicians and patients with prescribed medications. Am J Public Health 1976; 66(9):847–53.
[39] Kopjar B, Sales AE, Pineros SL, et al. Adherence with statin therapy in secondary prevention of coronary heart disease in Veterans Administration male population. Am J Cardiol 2003; 92(9):1106–8.
[40] Ellis JJ, Erickson SR, Stevenson JG, et al. Suboptimal statin adherence and discontinuation in primary and secondary prevention populations. J Gen Intern Med 2004;19(6):638–45.
[41] Gwadry-Sridhar FH, Arnold JM, Zhang Y, et al. Pilot study to determine the impact of a multidisciplinary educational intervention in patients hospitalized with heart failure. Am Heart J 2005;150(5):982.

[42] Jackson JE, Doescher MP, Saver BG, et al. Prescription drug coverage, health, and medication acquisition among seniors with one or more chronic conditions. Med Care 2004;42(11): 1056–65.

[43] Roe CM, Motheral BR, Teitelbaum F, et al. Angiotensin-converting enzyme inhibitor compliance and dosing among patients with heart failure. Am Heart J 1999;138(5 Pt 1):818–25.

[44] Cramer JA. Microelectronic systems for monitoring and enhancing patient compliance with medication regimens. Drugs 1995;49(3):321–7.

[45] Cheng CW, Woo KS, Chan JC, et al. Association between adherence to statin therapy and lipid control in Hong Kong Chinese patients at high risk of coronary heart disease. Br J Clin Pharmacol 2004;58(5):528–35.

[46] Dobbels F, De Geest S, van Cleemput J, et al. Effect of late medication non-compliance on outcome after heart transplantation: a 5-year follow-up. J Heart Lung Transplant 2004; 23(11):1245–51.

[47] Bouvy ML, Heerdink ER, Urquhart J, et al. Effect of a pharmacist-led intervention on diuretic compliance in heart failure patients: a randomized controlled study. J Card Fail 2003;9(5):404–11.

[48] Dunbar-Jacob J, Bohachick P, Mortimer MK, et al. Medication adherence in persons with cardiovascular disease. J Cardiovasc Nurs 2003;18(3):209–18.

[49] Chui MA, Deer M, Bennett SJ, et al. Association between adherence to diuretic therapy and health care utilization in patients with heart failure. Pharmacotherapy 2003;23(3):326–32.

[50] Leventhal MJ, Riegel B, Carlson B, et al. Negotiating compliance in heart failure: remaining issues and questions. Eur J Cardiovasc Nurs 2005;4(4):298–307.

[51] Happ MB, Naylor MD, Roe-Prior P. Factors contributing to rehospitalization of elderly patients with heart failure. J Cardiovasc Nurs 1997;11(4):75–84.

[52] Simpson SH, Farris KB, Johnson JA, et al. Using focus groups to identify barriers to drug use in patients with congestive heart failure. Pharmacotherapy 2000;20(7):823–9.

[53] Heszen-Klemens I, Lapinska E. Doctor-patient interaction, patients' health behavior and effects of treatment. Soc Sci Med 1984;19(1):9–18.

[54] Nagy VT, Wolfe GR. Cognitive predictors of compliance in chronic disease patients. Med Care 1984;22(10):912–21.

[55] Tolmie EP, Lindsay GM, Kerr SM, et al. Patients' perspectives on statin therapy for treatment of hypercholesterolaemia: a qualitative study. Eur J Cardiovasc Nurs 2003;2(2):141–9.

[56] Wiseman IC, Miller R. Quantifying non-compliance in patients receiving digoxin—a pharmacokinetic approach. S Afr Med J 1991;79(3):155–7.

[57] Schulz RM, Lingle EW, Chubon SJ, et al. Drug use behavior under the constraints of a Medicaid prescription cap. Clin Ther 1995;17(2):330–40.

[58] Hicks FD, Holm K. Self-management decision influences in heart failure: a preliminary investigation. Clin Nurs Res 2003;12(1):69–84.

[59] DiMatteo MR, Lepper HS, Croghan TW. Depression is a risk factor for noncompliance with medical treatment: meta-analysis of the effects of anxiety and depression on patient adherence. Arch Intern Med 2000;160(14):2101–7.

[60] Morgan AL, Masoudi FA, Havranek EP, et al. Difficulty taking medications, depression, and health status in heart failure patients. J Card Fail 2006;12(1):54–60.

[61] Carney RM, Freedland KE, Eisen SA, et al. Major depression and medication adherence in elderly patients with coronary artery disease. Health Psychol 1995;14(1):88–90.

[62] Wang PS, Bohn RL, Knight E, et al. Noncompliance with antihypertensive medications: the impact of depressive symptoms and psychosocial factors. J Gen Intern Med 2002;17(7): 504–11.

[63] Ziegelstein RC, Fauerbach JA, Stevens SS, et al. Patients with depression are less likely to follow recommendations to reduce cardiac risk during recovery from a myocardial infarction. Arch Intern Med 2000;160(12):1818–23.

[64] van der Wal MH, Jaarsma T, Moser DK, et al. Compliance in heart failure patients: the importance of knowledge and beliefs. Eur Heart J 2006;27(4):434–40.

[65] Senior V, Marteau TM, Weinman J. Self-reported adherence to cholesterol-lowering medication in patients with familial hypercholesterolaemia: the role of illness perceptions. Cardiovasc Drugs Ther 2004;18(6):475–81.

[66] Ohene Buabeng K, Matowe L, Plange-Rhule J. Unaffordable drug prices: the major cause of non-compliance with hypertension medication in Ghana. J Pharm Pharm Sci 2004;7(3): 350–2.

[67] Nikolaus T, Kruse W, Bach M, et al. Elderly patients' problems with medication. An in-hospital and follow-up study. Eur J Clin Pharmacol 1996;49(4):255–9.

[68] Riegel B, Carlson B. Facilitators and barriers to heart failure self-care. Patient Educ Couns 2002;46(4):287–95.

[69] Murray MD, Birt JA, Manatunga AK, et al. Medication compliance in elderly outpatients using twice-daily dosing and unit-of-use packaging. Ann Pharmacother 1993;27(5):616–21.

[70] George J, Shalansky SJ. Predictors of refill nonadherence in patients with heart failure. Br J Clin Pharmacol 2007;63(4):488–93.

[71] Lainscak M, Keber I. Patient's view of heart failure: from the understanding to the quality of life. Eur J Cardiovasc Nurs 2003;2(4):275–81.

[72] Agard A, Hermeren G, Herlitz J. When is a patient with heart failure adequately informed? A study of patients' knowledge of and attitudes toward medical information. Heart Lung 2004;33(4):219–26.

[73] DiMatteo MR. Social support and patient adherence to medical treatment: a meta-analysis. Health Psychol 2004;23(2):207–18.

[74] Schroeder K, Fahey T, Ebrahim S, et al. Adherence to long-term therapies: recent WHO report provides some answers but poses even more questions. J Clin Epidemiol 2004; 57(1):2–3.

[75] DiMatteo MR. Evidence-based strategies to foster adherence and improve patient outcomes. JAAPA 2004;17(11):18–21.

NURSING
CLINICS
OF NORTH AMERICA

ELSEVIER
SAUNDERS

Nurs Clin N Am 43 (2008) 155–170

Cognitive Behavioral Therapy for Depression in Patients with Heart Failure: A Critical Review

Rebecca L. Dekker, MSN, RN

College of Nursing, University of Kentucky, 760 Rose Street, Lexington, KY 40536-0232, USA

Depression is a significant problem in patients with heart failure (HF). One in five persons with HF has clinical depression [1], and up to 48% have clinically significant depressive symptoms [2]. According to the Diagnostic and Statistical Manual of Mental Disorders, Fourth Edition (DSM-IV-TR), a major depressive episode, sometimes referred to as clinical depression, consists of five or more symptoms which are present for most of the day, almost daily, for at least 2 weeks. One of these symptoms must be either depressed mood or loss of interest or pleasure in usual activities, and the symptoms must cause significant distress in social, occupational, or other areas of functioning (Box 1) [3]. However, patients can experience clinically significant depressive symptoms without the presence of a major depressive disorder [4]. Depressive symptoms may include depressed mood, irritability, guilt, hopelessness, low self-esteem, fatigue, sleep disturbances, appetite change, and inability to concentrate [5].

The adverse effects of clinical depression and depressive symptoms on mortality and hospitalizations in patients with HF have been well documented [1,2,6–8]. A recent meta-analysis demonstrated that patients with HF who have depressive symptoms are more than twice as likely to die or experience a cardiac event, when compared with patients without depressive symptoms [1]. Moreover, the presence of depressive symptoms has a negative impact on every aspect of health-related quality of life in patients with HF, including physical functioning, social functioning, and mental health [2].

Investigators must move beyond describing the problems associated with depression and depressive symptoms in patients with HF and begin to test interventions. There is a lack of research on nonpharmacologic interventions for depressive symptoms in patients with HF [9]. Cognitive behavioral therapy (CBT) has been used successfully to treat depression in multiple

E-mail address: rdekker@uky.edu

0029-6465/08/$ - see front matter © 2008 Elsevier Inc. All rights reserved.
doi:10.1016/j.cnur.2007.11.003
nursing.theclinics.com

Box 1. DSM-IV-TR criteria for a major depressive episode

At least five of the following symptoms have been present most
    of the day, nearly every day, during the same 2-week period
    and represent a change from previous functioning; at least one
    of the symptoms is either depressed mood or loss of interest or
    pleasure:

Depressed mood
Loss of interest or pleasure
Weight loss or changes in appetite
Insomnia or hypersomnia
Psychomotor agitation or retardation
Fatigue
Feelings of worthlessness or guilt
Decreased ability to concentrate
Thoughts of death, suicidal ideation, or suicide attempt

The symptoms must cause significant impairment in functioning
    (ie, work, social)
The symptoms must not be directly due to a medical condition
    (ie, hypothyroidism) or a medication
The episode is not better accounted for by a different diagnosis,
    such as bereavement, bipolar disorder, or schizoaffective
    disorder

Data from Diagnostic and statistical manual of mental disorders (DSM-IV-TR).
4th ed. Washington, D.C.: American Psychiatric Association, 2000.

---

populations [10,11]. Therefore, it may also be useful for treating depression
in patients with cardiovascular illnesses, including patients with HF. This article examines the empirical support for the use of CBT in treating depression
and depressive symptoms in patients with cardiovascular-related illnesses.

Background

   Aaron T. Beck, a psychiatrist, developed the Cognitive Model of depression in 1967. The model was developed to explain the psychologic processes
that occur in depression. The underlying assumption behind the Cognitive
Model was that human minds are biased and cannot interpret stimuli objectively. This bias leads to cognitive errors, or dysfunctional thinking [10]. The
Cognitive Model holds that dysfunctional thinking influences the emotions,
behaviors, and psychosomatic symptoms associated with depression. Thus,
interventions aimed at changing dysfunctional thinking should improve the
emotional, behavioral, and somatic symptoms of depression [11].

CBT is the psychotherapeutic intervention based on the Cognitive Model of depression. The primary goal of CBT is to alter emotions and behavior by redirecting negative cognitive processes. CBT is typically a short-term therapy that consists of 4 to 14 sessions, depending on the individual's progress. The role of the therapist is to develop a collaborative, therapeutic relationship with the client and to teach the client to become his or her own therapist. The therapist teaches the client to identify, analyze, and question dysfunctional thinking. For example, the therapist may help the client to identify negative thoughts, such as "I'm a burden to others." Together, the therapist and the client explore the evidence behind this negative thought. After evaluating the rationale for the thought, the therapist then guides the client to challenge the thought, and eventually change the client's thinking. By creating changes in thinking, the client may modify negative emotions and behaviors [11].

CBT offers several potential advantages for the treatment of depression and depressive symptoms in patients with HF. First, CBT is a nonpharmacologic intervention. Nonpharmacologic interventions may have several advantages over pharmacologic treatments, such as a lack of drug-drug interactions, immediate short-term relief of symptoms, and greater involvement of patients in their own self-care. Second, CBT is an intervention that nurses can be trained to administer. CBT is compatible with common nursing interventions of teaching patients to accurately appraise stressors, determining the best coping method, and increasing perceived control. Despite the potential benefits of CBT, its effectiveness in patients with cardiovascular illness, including HF, remains unknown. The following review provides a critical analysis of the existing research on the effectiveness of CBT for treating depression or depressive symptoms in patients with cardiovascular illnesses.

Methods

The databases searched for relevant literature were PUBMED, PsychInfo, CINAHL, and MEDLINE. Keywords included "depress*" and "cognitive behavioral therapy" (or cognitive therapy) and "cardiovascular" (or heart failure, chronic illness, coronary artery disease, cardiac, stroke, or diabetes). The search was limited to English language articles published between 1980 and 2007. Studies were included in the review if they met the following criteria: randomized, controlled trial (RCT), a cognitive behavioral intervention, depression or depressive symptoms measured as an outcome, and samples consisted of patients with cardiovascular disease, nonhemorrhagic stroke, or type II diabetes. Diabetes mellitus commonly coexists with HF [12] and is an important risk factor for the development of HF [13]. Thus, samples that contained patients with type II diabetes were also included. The search resulted in 331 studies of which the titles or abstracts were screened for inclusion criteria. Reference lists of relevant articles were screened for additional studies. A total of ten papers met the inclusion criteria and were extracted for review.

Results

Cardiovascular disease

Six studies were identified in which the impact of CBT on depression in patients with cardiovascular disease was evaluated (Table 1). In the largest randomized controlled trial on CBT in cardiovascular disease to date, the Enhancing Recovery in Coronary Heart Disease (ENRICHD) investigators [14] compared the impact of CBT with usual care on depressive symptoms and event-free survival in 2,481 subjects with a recent myocardial infarction (MI). Patients were eligible to participate if they were defined as depressed on a diagnostic interview or if they had low perceived social support. The intervention consisted of CBT in conjunction with selective serotonin reuptake inhibitor when indicated.

The investigators found that the intervention group experienced a statistically significant decrease in depressive symptoms, compared with the control group, at 6 months. However, this difference was no longer present at 30 or 42 months of follow-up. There was no difference in event-free survival between the intervention and control groups. The lack of impact on event-free survival may have been a result of several factors. The ENRICHD investigators assumed that CBT should begin as soon as possible (within 28 days) after an MI. Thus, the study may have included patients in the control group who had transient rather than clinical depression and recovered without intervention. The investigators also assumed that the usual care group would not receive treatment for depression, but this was not the case. Antidepressant use reached 21% in the control group and 28% in the intervention group [14–16]. It is not known why a decrease in depressive symptoms in the intervention group in this study did not translate into improved outcomes. It may be that the decrease in depressive symptoms was insufficient to affect clinical outcomes. This conclusion is supported by the observation that, while depressive symptoms in the intervention group decreased by 49%, depressive symptoms in the control group also decreased by 33% [14].

Twenty years ago, Burgess and colleagues [17] reported that an intervention combining CBT, social support, and job return counseling failed to reduce depressive symptoms in patients who had recently experienced an acute MI. In this randomized, controlled trial, 180 subjects were randomized to the intervention group or usual care. There were no differences in depression scores between groups at baseline, 3 months, or 13 months of follow-up. The investigators did not offer any possible explanations for the null effects on depression. Females were underrepresented in the study; thus, it is not known whether the intervention would have been ineffective for females as well.

CBT may be effective in reducing depressive symptoms in survivors of sudden cardiac death. Cowan and colleagues [18,19] tested the impact of CBT, biofeedback therapy, and health education on depressive symptoms and mortality in 133 survivors of sudden cardiac death. Only 11% of the sample had depressive symptoms at baseline, and all of the participants with depressive symptoms were male. Approximately half of the sample had chronic heart failure (New York Heart Association [NYHA] Functional Class II–IV). The treatment group experienced a significant decrease in depressive symptoms compared with the control group. Although the study was not powered to detect differences in mortality, the treatment group experienced an 86% reduction in the risk of cardiac death when compared with the control group. Therefore, the results of this study suggest that CBT and biofeedback may be beneficial for survivors of sudden cardiac death, whether or not they are experiencing depressive symptoms.

Limited evidence suggests that CBT may be more effective than exercise at reducing depressive symptoms in patients with coronary artery disease. Black and colleagues [20] randomized 60 subjects who had recently been hospitalized for a coronary event and were psychologically distressed to one of two groups: a special intervention that consisted of stress management, relaxation training, and CBT administered by a psychiatrist, or a cardiac rehabilitation group that included exercise and risk reduction counseling. At 6 months, the CBT group experienced a significant reduction in depressive symptoms, compared with the cardiac rehabilitation group. There was no difference between groups with regard to rehospitalizations. There were several limitations of the study, such as low representation of women (12%), exclusion of elderly (over 80 years old), and lack of a true control group. Most importantly, adherence to the intervention was low. Less than 50% of participants attended more than one intervention session. Crossover between groups was also a problem, as six participants in the usual care group were treated with antidepressants or psychologic counseling. Combined, these limitations severely weakened the internal and external validity of the study.

There is some evidence to suggest that CBT may be helpful for reducing depressive symptoms in patients with implanted cardioverter defibrillators (ICDs). Frizelle and colleagues [21] compared the impact of a cardiac rehabilitation and CBT to a wait list control group on depressive symptoms in patients with ICDs. Despite the small sample size (n = 22), the intervention group experienced a significant reduction in depressive symptoms when compared with the control group at 3 months. The intervention included exercise, which makes it impossible to ascertain whether the CBT alone had an impact on depressive symptoms.

In another study, Kohn and colleagues [22] evaluated the effects of CBT on depressive symptoms in 49 subjects with ICDs. This study was limited by the lack of a comprehensive measure of depressive symptoms at baseline. Only three biologic indicators of depression were measured at

Table 1
Study characteristics and findings

First author (year)	Design and follow-up time	Sample	Measurement of depression	Treatment	Control	Results
Berkman [14] (2003)	RCT Two arms 30 months	n = 2,481 28 days post-MI Eligible if classified as depressed or low perceived social support Females 44% Minorities 34%	DISH, BDI, HRSD	11 tailored CBT sessions over 6 months, group therapy as needed, referral to psychiatry for antidepressants as needed	Usual care; physicians were notified if patients were depressed or had low perceived social support	The CBT group had a lower BDI score compared with control (9.1 versus 12.2, $P < .001$), and a lower HRSD score (7.6 versus 9.4, $P < .001$) at 6 months. This difference was not present at 30 or 42 months.
Burgess [17] (1987)	RCT Two arms 13 months	n = 180 Post acute MI Females 14% Minorities not reported	ZDS	A mean of 6.32 CBT visits per patient, social support, facilitation of job return	Usual care	There were no differences between groups on depression scores at baseline or follow-up
Cowan [18,19] (2001)	RCT Two arms 3 months	n = 133 Sudden cardiac death survivors Females 27% Minorities 10%	SCR-90: Depression subscale	11 sessions of combined CBT, biofeedback, and health education, administered biweekly for 6 weeks	90-minute health education class	Depressive symptoms decreased in the treatment group when compared with the control group

Study	Design	Sample	Measure	Intervention	Control	Results
Black [20] (1998)	RCT Two arms 6 months	n = 60 Recently hospitalized for angina, MI, angioplasty, or CABG Eligible if scored as distressed Females 12% Minorities not reported	SCR-90: Depression subscale	1 to 7 weekly sessions with a psychologist including: relaxation training, stress management, reduction of risk factors, efforts to improve adherence, and CBT intervention; antidepressants if necessary	Cardiac rehabilitation with monitored exercise one to three times per week, for 8 weeks, daily home exercise. Education on stress management, support group meeting with spouses, individual nutrition counseling	The CBT group had significant reductions in depressive symptoms compared with the control group (-5.2 versus -0.2, $P < .034$)
Frizelle [21] (2004)	RCT Two arms 3 months	n = 22 Patients with ICDs Females not reported Minorities not reported	HADS	Group-based therapy, 6 sessions, 1 hour each: home-based exercise, education, relaxation, behavioral goal setting, education on identifying and challenging negative thoughts	Wait-list	The treatment group experienced decreases in depressive symptoms compared with the control group (-4.25 versus -0.2, $P = .001$)
Kohn [22] (2000)	RCT Two arms 9 months	n = 49 Post ICD implantation Females 35% African American 8%	BDI version II; four biologic measures of depression: sexual functioning, appetite, weight change, and sleep patterns	9 sessions ranging from 15–90 minutes, sessions included psycho-education on: anxieties about ICD, avoidance behavior, fear of shocks, stress management, work and social activities, distorted cognitions	Usual care	The CBT group had lower levels of depressive symptoms at follow-up compared with the control group (6.9 versus 15, $P = .037$), but depressive symptoms were not measured at baseline

(continued on next page)

Table 1 (*continued*)

First author (year)	Design and follow-up time	Sample	Measurement of depression	Treatment	Control	Results
Kostis [23] (1994)	RCT Three arms 3 months	n = 20 Patients with congestive heart failure Female 30% Minorities not reported	BDI	12 weeks of exercise training at a cardiac rehab facility for 1 hour three times per week; weekly meetings with a dietician; group-based CBT intervention: twice weekly for 60–90 min (relaxation, positive imagery, appraisal of negative cognitions)	1. Lanoxin titrated to achieve levels between 0.8–2.0 ng/mL 2. Placebo	There was a 52% decrease in BDI scores in the intervention group compared with a 15% and 25% increase in the control groups at follow up ($P = .04$)
Lincoln [24] (2003)	RCT Three arms 6 months	n = 123 1–6 months post CVA Eligible if scored as depressed Female 49% Minorities not reported	BDI WDI	10 1-hour sessions over 3 months, tailored CBT intervention: education, task assignment, activity scheduling, identification and modification of inaccurate thoughts	1. No intervention 2. Attention placebo: ten 1 hour visits over 3 months	No significant differences between groups in depression scores

Lustman [25] (1998)	RCT Two arms 6 months	n = 51 Type II diabetes and major depression Females 60% Minorities 19%	DIS BDI	1 hour/week of individual CBT for 10 weeks, strategies included: behavioral strategies, problem solving, and cognitive techniques to change cognitive errors	Attention placebo: 1 hour, biweekly, individual sessions with a diabetes educator	The CBT group had a higher rate of remission from depression compared with the control group (58.3% versus 25.9%, $P = .03$)
Henry [26] (1997)	RCT Two arms 7 weeks	n = 19 Type II diabetes Females 53% Minorities not reported	BDI	6 sessions of 1.5 hours per: progressive muscle relaxation, cognitive coping training (such as identifying and modifying negative thoughts), problem-solving skills, homework assignments	Wait-list	Depressive symptoms decreased across time in both groups; there was no difference between groups

Abbreviations: BDI, Beck Depression Inventory version I; CVA, cardiovascular accident; CABG, coronary-artery bypass grafting surgery; DIS, diagnostic interview schedule; DISH, Depression Interview and Structured Hamilton; HADS, Hospital Anxiety & Depression Scale; HRSD, Hamilton Rating Scale for Depression; ICD, implanted cardioverter defibrillators; MI, myocardial infarction; SCR-90, Symptom checklist 90 revised; WDI, Wakefield Depression Inventory; ZDS, Zung Depression Scale.

baseline: sexual functioning difficulties, changes in appetite, and sleep disturbance. At 9 months follow-up, the CBT group reported fewer sexual functioning difficulties than the control group; however, sexual difficulties
increased in both groups over time. The Beck Depression Inventory II
(BDI-II) was administered only at follow-up. Although the CBT group
had a lower BDI-II score than the control group at follow-up, the lack of
depression score data at baseline limits the conclusions that can be drawn
from the findings.

Finally, results from a small study suggest that an intense regimen of
CBT combined with exercise may reduce depressive symptoms in patients
with HF [23]. In this study, 20 subjects with HF (NYHA Class II or III)
were randomized to three groups: group-based CBT plus exercise, Digoxin
titrated to achieve drug levels between 0.8 to 2.0 ng/mL, or placebo. Despite
the small sample size, the intervention group experienced a 52% reduction
in depressive symptoms, while the other groups experienced a 15% and
25% increase in depressive symptoms, respectively. The interpretation of
findings from this study is limited by the combination of exercise with
CBT. It is not known whether CBT alone would have been effective in
decreasing depressive symptoms. In addition, the follow-up period was
short, only 12 weeks, and therefore no conclusions can be drawn regarding
the long-term effects of the intervention.

Stroke

There is less evidence regarding the effectiveness of CBT on depression in
patients with stroke. Lincoln and Flannaghan [24] conducted a randomized,
controlled trial in which 123 subjects who had recently experienced a stroke
and experienced depressive symptoms (scored more than 10 on the BDI)
were assigned to one of three groups: CBT, an attention placebo group,
or a control group. Surprisingly, depressive symptoms improved over time
in all of the groups. There were no significant differences among the groups
at baseline, 3 months, and 6 months of follow-up. The investigators suggest
that the intervention, which consisted of ten 1-hour sessions, may not have
been intense enough to improve depressive symptoms more than would
occur naturally. However, other investigators have tested CBT in chronic
illness and found positive results using a similar number of CBT sessions
[14,25]. It is possible that the improvement in depressive symptoms in all
three groups over time may have reflected the natural improvement of
depression that occurs over time after an acute stroke [24].

Diabetes

The effectiveness of CBT for the management of depression in patients
with type II diabetes has only been tested in two RCTs. Lustman and
colleagues [25] conducted an RCT in which 51 subjects with diabetes
and clinical depression were assigned to either 10 weeks of CBT and

diabetes education or an education-only group. As a result of the intervention, the treatment group had a higher rate of remission from depression when compared with the control group (58.3% versus 25.9%). In contrast, Henry and colleagues [26] found that CBT did not improve depressive symptoms in patients with type II diabetes. This small RCT evaluated the effects of progressive muscle relaxation and CBT on depressive symptoms in 19 subjects with type II diabetes who had elevated levels of glycosylated hemoglobin. Although there was an overall decrease in depressive symptoms from pretreatment to posttreatment, there was no difference between groups. Because of the small sample size, the study was likely under-powered to detect changes in depressive symptoms between groups.

Discussion

Ten randomized, controlled trials were identified in which investigators tested the impact of CBT on depression or depressive symptoms in patients with cardiovascular-related illnesses. Although positive effects were reported in six of the ten studies regarding the impact of CBT on depression or depressive symptoms, many of the studies had limitations that weakened internal or external validity. The major factors that contributed to the mixed results were:

- More than one intervention was tested in most studies
- The interventions were not described adequately, making replication difficult
- There was a lack of a true, no-intervention control group in most studies
- Most had small sample sizes
- Follow-up periods were short
- Women were underrepresented
- A variety of instruments were used to measure depressive symptoms
- There was a lack of adherence to the Consolidated Standards of Reporting Trials (CONSORT) guidelines for the reporting of clinical trials

The presence of more than one treatment in the intervention of several studies restricts the ability to determine the effect of CBT on outcomes. In two studies, CBT and antidepressant therapy were combined [14,20], making it impossible to determine the effect of CBT alone on depressive symptoms. Similarly, in two other studies, the intervention consisted of CBT plus exercise [21,23]. A growing body of evidence has demonstrated that exercise is an effective treatment for persons with major depressive disorders or with depressive symptoms [27,28]. Thus, exercise in combination with CBT may have yielded a larger effect than CBT alone, or may obscure the effect of CBT. In addition, the CBT interventions used were often described vaguely. It may be possible that the investigators tested different forms of CBT, which could contribute to the mixed findings. Furthermore, by incompletely describing the intervention, future replication and verification of the results is made difficult.

Lack of a true, no-intervention group was present in four of the ten studies reviewed. These studies included a variety of comparison groups. One group of investigators compared the CBT intervention to a group that received an exercise intervention [20]. The comparison of CBT to exercise may yield a small or insignificant effect, given that both can decrease depressive symptoms. The inclusion of a third, true control group, would have allowed investigators to compare the effects of CBT with exercise.

With the exception of the ENRICHD trial, all of the studies had small sample sizes and a relatively short follow-up period. Sample sizes in nine studies ranged from 19 to 180, and follow-up periods ranged from 7 weeks to 13 months. Despite the ENRICHD trial's large sample size and long follow-up period, the investigators found only modest clinically significant reductions in depressive symptoms. Moreover, this benefit was no longer present by 30 months of follow-up [14]. In contrast, smaller studies found that CBT did reduce depressive symptoms at a relatively short follow-up time. It is possible that the improvements in depressive symptoms found in these studies did not persist. Short follow-up times limit the ability of researchers to determine whether CBT is an effective long-term treatment for depression.

Six of the ten studies had samples that consisted of at least 30% women. Of these six studies, three found that CBT reduced depressive symptoms. Previous research has demonstrated that women may react differently to psychologic interventions than men. In a post-hoc analysis, the ENRICHD investigators reported that white men who received the CBT intervention had a reduced risk of experiencing cardiac mortality or recurrent MI. In contrast, there was no such beneficial effect for women and minorities [29]. Frasure-Smith and colleagues [30] reported that women who received an intense psychosocial nursing intervention after an MI experienced an increase in all-cause mortality when compared with the control group (10.3% versus 5.4%). This adverse effect was not found in the male participants. The results of these two studies suggest that it is important to evaluate the impact of psychologic interventions on both men and women. Overall, the studies in this review provide insufficient evidence to determine the impact of CBT on depressive symptoms in women with cardiovascular illness.

A definition of depression or depressive symptoms was not provided in a majority of the studies. Depression has been referred to as "a notoriously slippery word, simultaneously connoting states that range from mild, transient unhappiness to life-threatening, catatonic stupors" [31]. In this review, some researchers referred to clinical depression, depression, and depressive symptoms interchangeably, without clarifying the meaning. Researchers also used a variety of methods to measure clinical depression and depressive symptoms. Many of these measures, such as the Beck Depression Inventory, have established reliability and validity. In contrast, Kohn and colleagues

[22] used an instrument that measured three biologic indicators of depression. The reliability and validity of this instrument was not provided. Overall, there was a lack of consistency on the measurement of depression in the reviewed studies. This limitation may contribute to the mixed findings of this review.

The CONSORT guidelines were originally published in 1996 and have since been revised [32,33]. These guidelines provide a standardized framework for the reporting of clinical trials. Of the eight studies that were published after 1996, only two followed the CONSORT guidelines [14,24]. The CONSORT guidelines allow the reader to understand the design, conduct, analysis, and interpretation of an RCT, and to judge whether a trial has internal or external validity [33]. The lack of adherence to the CONSORT guidelines exhibited by some of the reviewed studies makes it difficult to interpret the results and determine validity.

Implications for nursing research

The problems associated with depression and depressive symptoms in patients with HF have been adequately described. Studies testing interventions for treating depression in patients with HF are now needed to move us toward development of effective nonpharmacologic treatment. CBT has been shown to be effective in treating depression in other populations. However, the current evidence to support CBT as a treatment for depression or depressive symptoms in patients with cardiovascular-related illnesses is inconclusive because of limitations of existing studies.

Based on this review, future clinical trials should include the following recommendations. Investigators should test the effect of a CBT intervention alone, as well as in combination with other treatments. The CBT intervention should be replicable in a clinical setting. Careful consideration should be paid to the inclusion of an appropriate comparison group. Given that depression in patients with HF is associated with a high risk for morbidity and mortality, it may be unethical to withhold treatment for depression from patients who are known to be clinically depressed. Perhaps investigators should exclude patients with diagnosed clinical depression and instead refer them to their primary care providers for treatment.

Studies should be designed to have large enough sample sizes to be adequately powered to detect changes in depressive symptoms and related outcomes. Investigators should also make special efforts to include a representative sample of women. In addition, trials should include an adequate follow-up time of at least one year to provide information on the long-term effectiveness of CBT. It is also important that investigators use consistent methods for measuring depressive symptoms. In 2006, the National Heart, Lung, and Blood Institute issued recommendations regarding the measurement of depression in cardiovascular research. The recommendations state that depression severity rating during a trial should be measured by the Beck Depression Inventory, the Inventory of Depressive Symptoms, or the Hamilton Rating Scale for Depression [34]. Finally, investigators should follow the CONSORT guidelines [33] in the reporting of their RCTs.

Several gaps in the understanding of CBT as a treatment for depression in cardiovascular illness remain. It is not known if there is a dose-response relationship between CBT and depression in patients with cardiovascular disease. The best time to intervene for depressive symptoms in patients with cardiovascular disease is also unknown. Patients with HF who are hospitalized are extremely vulnerable to depressive symptoms, and 60% of these patients still have depressive symptoms 1 year after discharge [35]. The results of the ENRICHD trial showed that patients who had recently experienced a cardiac event and received a CBT intervention only experienced a minimal improvement in depressive symptoms. This led investigators to question whether CBT should be offered to patients who have recently experienced a cardiac event, or if treatment should be delayed [15]. Next, it is not known whether CBT interventions should be offered only to patients with HF who are clinically depressed or to all patients with HF, regardless of depression. Finally, it is unknown whether CBT can affect outcomes related to depression, such as mortality, morbidity, or health-related quality of life in patients with cardiovascular illness.

Implications for nursing practice

CBT is compatible with nursing practice and has been used successfully to treat depression in medically healthy populations. The current evidence, however, is insufficient to recommend CBT as a treatment for depressive symptoms in patients with cardiovascular illness. Although the majority of the studies reviewed demonstrated that CBT may be effective, the limitations in study design prevent wide generalization of the results. More studies need to be conducted before nurses should routinely refer patients with cardiovascular illness to CBT for the treatment of depression or depressive symptoms. It is important to also note that CBT may not be appropriate for all patients with HF or cardiovascular illness, particularly for patients who may have difficulty adhering to the CBT treatment protocol. These patients may benefit from alternative treatments for depression.

Summary

Depression is a significant clinical problem in patients with HF. The time has come for investigators to focus their efforts on designing and testing nonpharmacologic interventions for depression in patients with HF. Cognitive behavioral therapy holds promise as an intervention that may decrease depressive symptoms in patients with cardiovascular illness, including heart failure. Nurses should continue to monitor the literature for new evidence regarding the effectiveness of CBT for treating depression in patients with HF and other cardiovascular illnesses.

Acknowledgment

The author would like to acknowledge Dr. Susan K. Frazier, Dr. Terry A. Lennie, and Dr. Debra K. Moser at the University of Kentucky for their mentorship during the writing of this article.

References

[1] Rutledge T, Reis VA, Linke SE, et al. Depression in heart failure: a meta-analytic review of prevalence, intervention effects, and associations with clinical outcomes. J Am Coll Cardiol 2006;48(8):1527–37.

[2] Gottlieb SS, Khatta M, Friedmann E, et al. The influence of age, gender, and race on the prevalence of depression in heart failure patients. J Am Coll Cardiol 2004;43(9):1542–9.

[3] American Psychiatric Association. Diagnostic and statistical manual of mental disorders (DSM-IV-TR). 4th edition. Washington, DC: American Psychiatric Association; 2000.

[4] Judd LL, Akiskal HS, Zeller PJ, et al. Psychosocial disability during the long-term course of unipolar major depressive disorder. Arch Gen Psychiatry 2000;57(4):375–80.

[5] Stuart GW. Emotional responses and mood disorders. In: Stuart GW, Laraia MT, editors. Principles and practice of psychiatric nursing, Vol. 7th editionSt. Louis (MO): Mosby; 2001. p. 345–80.

[6] Jiang W, Kuchibhatla M, Clary GL, et al. Relationship between depressive symptoms and long-term mortality in patients with heart failure. Am Heart J 2007;154(1):102–8.

[7] Faris R, Purcell H, Henein MY, et al. Clinical depression is common and significantly associated with reduced survival in patients with non-ischaemic heart failure. Eur J Heart Fail 2002;4(4):541–51.

[8] Jiang W, Alexander J, Christopher E, et al. Relationship of depression to increased risk of mortality and rehospitalization in patients with congestive heart failure. Arch Intern Med 2001;161(15):1849–56.

[9] Lane DA, Chong AY, Lip GY. Psychological interventions for depression in heart failure. Cochrane Database Syst Rev 2005;(1):CD003329.

[10] Beck AT. The current state of cognitive therapy: a 40-year retrospective. Arch Gen Psychiatry 2005;62(9):953–9.

[11] Beck JS. Cognitive therapy: basics and beyond. New York: Guilford Press; 1995.

[12] Masoudi FA, Inzucchi SE. Diabetes mellitus and heart failure: epidemiology, mechanisms, and pharmacotherapy. Am J Cardiol 2007;99(4A):113B–32B.

[13] Levy D, Larson MG, Vasan RS, et al. The progression from hypertension to congestive heart failure. JAMA 1996;275(20):1557–62.

[14] Berkman LF, Blumenthal J, Burg M, et al. Effects of treating depression and low perceived social support on clinical events after myocardial infarction: the Enhancing Recovery in Coronary Heart Disease Patients (ENRICHD) Randomized Trial. JAMA 2003;289(23):3106–16.

[15] Joynt KE, O'Connor CM. Lessons from SADHART, ENRICHD, and other trials. Psychosom Med 2005;(67 Suppl 1):S63–6.

[16] Frasure-Smith N, Lesperance F. Depression—a cardiac risk factor in search of a treatment. JAMA 2003;289(23):3171–3.

[17] Burgess AW, Lerner DJ, D'Agostino RB, et al. A randomized control trial of cardiac rehabilitation. Soc Sci Med 1987;24(4):359–70.

[18] Cowan MJ, Pike KC, Budzynski HK. Psychosocial nursing therapy following sudden cardiac arrest: impact on two-year survival. Nurs Res 2001;50(2):68–76.

[19] Cowan MJ. Innovative approaches: a psychosocial therapy for sudden cardiac arrest survivors. In: Dunbar SB, Ellenbogen KA, Epstein AE, editors. Sudden cardiac death: past, present, and future. Armonk (NY): Futura Publishing Company, Inc; 1997. p. 371–86.

[20] Black JL, Allison TG, Williams DE, et al. Effect of intervention for psychological distress on rehospitalization rates in cardiac rehabilitation patients. Psychosomatics 1998;39(2):134–43.

[21] Frizelle DJ, Lewin RJ, Kaye G, et al. Cognitive-behavioural rehabilitation programme for patients with an implanted cardioverter defibrillator: a pilot study. Br J Health Psychol 2004;9(Pt 3):381–92.

[22] Kohn CS, Petrucci RJ, Baessler C, et al. The effect of psychological intervention on patients' long-term adjustment to the ICD: a prospective study. Pacing Clin Electrophysiol 2000;23 (4 Pt 1):450–6.

[23] Kostis JB, Rosen RC, Cosgrove NM, et al. Nonpharmacologic therapy improves functional and emotional status in congestive heart failure. Chest 1994;106(4):996–1001.

[24] Lincoln NB, Flannaghan T. Cognitive behavioral psychotherapy for depression following stroke: a randomized controlled trial. Stroke 2003;34(1):111–5.

[25] Lustman PJ, Griffith LS, Freedland KE, et al. Cognitive behavior therapy for depression in type 2 diabetes mellitus: a randomized, controlled trial. Ann Intern Med 1998;129(8):613–21.

[26] Henry JL, Wilson PH, Bruce DG, et al. Cognitive-behavioural stress management for patients with non-insulin dependent diabetes mellitus. Psychol Health Med 1997;2(2): 109–18.

[27] Blumenthal JA, Babyak MA, Moore KA, et al. Effects of exercise training on older patients with major depression. Arch Intern Med 1999;159(19):2349–56.

[28] Dunn AL, Trivedi MH, Kampert JB, et al. Exercise treatment for depression: efficacy and dose response. Am J Prev Med 2005;28(1):1–8.

[29] Schneiderman N, Saab PG, Catellier DJ, et al. Psychosocial treatment within sex by ethnicity subgroups in the Enhancing Recovery in Coronary Heart Disease clinical trial. Psychosom Med 2004;66(4):475–83.

[30] Frasure-Smith N, Lesperance F, Prince RH, et al. Randomised trial of home-based psychosocial nursing intervention for patients recovering from myocardial infarction. Lancet 1997;350(9076):473–9.

[31] Raison CL, Purselle DC, Capuron L, et al. Treatment of depression in medical illness. In: Licinio J, Wong ML, editors. Biology of Depression: From Novel Insights to Therapeutic Strategies, Vol. 1Weinheim (Germany): Wiley-VCH; 2005. p. 253–78.

[32] Begg C, Cho M, Eastwood S, et al. Improving the quality of reporting of randomized controlled trials. The CONSORT statement. JAMA 1996;276(8):637–9.

[33] Moher D, Schulz KF, Altman D. The CONSORT statement: revised recommendations for improving the quality of reports of parallel-group randomized trials. JAMA 2001;285(15): 1987–91.

[34] Davidson KW, Kupfer DJ, Bigger JT, et al. Assessment and treatment of depression in patients with cardiovascular disease: National Heart, Lung, and Blood Institute working group report. Ann Behav Med 2006;32(2):121–6.

[35] Koenig HG. Depression in hospitalized older patients with congestive heart failure. Gen Hosp Psychiatry 1998;20(1):29–43.

ELSEVIER
SAUNDERS

Nurs Clin N Am 43 (2008) 171–177

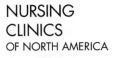

NURSING
CLINICS
OF NORTH AMERICA

Index

Note: Page numbers of article titles are in **boldface** type.

0029-6465/08/$ - see front matter © 2008 Elsevier Inc. All rights reserved.
doi:10.1016/S0029-6465(07)00093-X

nursing.theclinics.com

Moving?

Make sure your subscription moves with you!

To notify us of your new address, find your **Clinics Account Number** (located on your mailing label above your name), and contact customer service at:

E-mail: elspcs@elsevier.com

800-654-2452 (subscribers in the U.S. & Canada)
407-345-4000 (subscribers outside of the U.S. & Canada)

Fax number: 407-363-9661

Elsevier Periodicals Customer Service
6277 Sea Harbor Drive
Orlando, FL 32887-4800

*To ensure uninterrupted delivery of your subscription, please notify us at least 4 weeks in advance of move.